A Pharmacist's Guide to Inpatient Medical Emergencies

Pharmacy Joe
Joseph Muench PharmD, BCPS

Published by
RxJ Solutions, LLC

Visit:
pharmacyjoe.com

The author and publisher of this work have made every effort to provide information that is accurate and complete at the time of publication. However in view of the possibility of human error or changes in medical sciences, neither the author nor publisher warrants that the information contained herein is in every aspect accurate or complete, and they disclaim all responsibility for any errors or omissions, or for the results obtained from the use of the information contained in this work. Readers are encouraged to confirm the information contained herein with other sources. For example and in particular, readers are advised to check the product information sheet included in the package of each medication they plan to recommend, dispense, or administer to be certain that the information contained in this work is accurate and that changes have not been made in the recommended dose or in the contraindications for administration.

Comments or suggestions? Click or visit:

pharmacyjoe.com/contact

To

My family, for your endless support and love.

About the Author

Pharmacy Joe is a husband, father, critical care pharmacist, podcaster, author, and founder of pharmacyjoe.com where he provides valuable, unbiased critical care pharmacy content.

Tune in to hear Pharmacy Joe's #1 ranked critical care pharmacy podcast: The Elective Rotation. You can find the show in iTunes, Stitcher, or by going to: pharmacyjoe.com

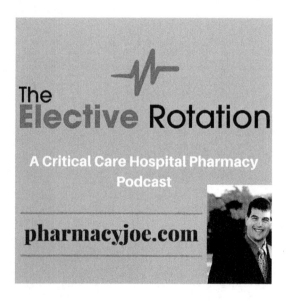

How To Use This Book

Thank you for purchasing a copy of *A Pharmacist's Guide to Inpatient Medical Emergencies*. This book is written to help pharmacists learn and refine the clinical skill of responding to *adult* inpatient medical emergencies.

PART I
Chapters 1 through 3 detail how to respond *in general* to inpatient medical emergencies. These chapters provide actionable suggestions for responding to code blue and rapid response calls, patient assessment, and verbal communication with physicians / providers.

PART II
Chapters 4 through 21 detail how to respond *to specific* inpatient medical emergencies. Each chapter covers a single emergency and has a standard format:

KEY POINTS
At the beginning of each chapter, there is a brief overview of the essential steps necessary to manage the emergency. This section is designed to be a quick reference that can be consulted during an emergency.

OBSERVATIONS
This section describes what you would expect to see if a patient was experiencing the emergency.

INTERVENTIONS
This section details specific treatments for each emergency.

ADDITIONAL SECTIONS
Additional sections may include "Preparations" if there is a significant amount of preparing to be done (such as in endotracheal intubation) and "Complications" to detail what to expect if the emergency is not initially managed successfully.

REFERENCES
This section includes supporting evidence as well as suggested readings for further information.

This book assumes that the reader has a working knowledge of Advanced Cardiac Life Support guidelines as well as a tertiary reference for complete information on medication contraindications, warnings, and adverse reactions.

Contents

PART I

Chapter 1

Introduction to Emergency Response

In 2007, I joined my hospital's medical emergency team. At the time, I was very nervous! Nothing in my pharmacy training or career prepared me for responding to medical emergencies. I was concerned that I would not have a role on the team - they had gotten by for years without a pharmacist, what could they possibly need one for? I was wondering what heroic or fantastic thing I would have to do to fit in or prove my worth to the team.

Over the years, I have become increasingly comfortable and confident in my role on the hospital medical emergency team. I have trained many of my colleagues and PGY-1 residents on the vital role a pharmacist has when responding to *adult* inpatient medical emergencies. This book contains the information that I wish was available to me when I first joined the team years ago.

Let's dive in:

Arriving at the emergency

Take the stairs when possible to reach the site of the emergency. The elevator can be frustratingly slow. The following Twitter poll was in favor of taking the stairs by a 2:1 margin:

Pharmacy Joe @PharmacyJoe · Jun 11
An inpatient code blue is called 5 floors above you. **What is** the best way to get there? #FOAMed

68% Stairs

32% Elevator

98 votes · Final results

When you enter the room, identify your role to staff already in attendance ("I'm a pharmacist" or "Pharmacy is here").

Carefully observe the patient and the care being administered:

Are chest compressions being performed?
What does the patient look like? Respiratory distress?
Unresponsive? Alert?
What are the patient's vital signs?
What other team members are present?

Do not be hesitant

The number one thing that holds back pharmacists from successfully responding to medical emergencies is hesitation to be involved in the emergency scenario. You can not help the patient or the team if you are out in the hallway or standing silently against the wall.

It is completely normal to be nervous or to lack confidence as you begin responding to medical emergencies. While this book will help you acquire the knowledge you need to respond to medical emergencies, it is up to YOU to put yourself side-by-side with the rest of the team so that you can gain experience and confidence.

Be a pharmacist

The knowledge and skill you have from your training as a pharmacist is what makes you valuable to the patient and team during a medical emergency. In many cases, you do not need to do anything different than if you were working in the IV room in the central pharmacy.

When you take responsibility for the pharmacotherapy needs of the patient, you are allowing other team members (nurse, physician / provider) to be hands-on with the patient.

You are providing a valuable service to the patient and team even if 'all you are doing' is calculating doses, preparing and labeling medications, or answering compatibility questions. With the experience and confidence you gain over time, you will provide additional value by helping to identify and reverse the cause(s) of the patient's clinical deterioration.

An emergency scenario will be a faster pace than you may be used to. Instead of working or thinking at a faster pace (which could lead to errors), prepare in advance for the needs of the patient and team. By anticipating pharmacotherapy needs in advance, you can keep up with the fast pace of an emergency scenario without sacrificing safety.

Label medications

Properly labeled syringes and IV lines will help prevent medication errors. You will need to prepare labels ahead of time so you do not slow down the administration of critical medications.

Keep preprinted labels in your medication boxes and / or a roll of medical tape in your lab coat to label syringes and IV lines. In a pinch, you can always tape the syringe and medication vial together.

As the IV drips start to pile up, it can be very confusing and time consuming for the nurse to sort them out. By labeling the IV lines, you can facilitate the nurse getting the right medications to the patient and working around IV incompatibilities. Place a label near the port closest to the patient and another label on the section of tubing that is above the smart pump.

Be sure to include the medication name, the date, and time the IV infusion was hung on the label so the nurse can change the tubing at the appropriate time.

Provide medications in the most ready to administer form

For IV infusions, this means to prime IV tubing (have a nurse show you) and label the lines.

For IV push medications, give the nurse a primed saline flush and an alcohol swab along with a labeled syringe of the medications.

Facilitate obtaining medications from the central pharmacy

When an unconventional therapy is needed to help the patient (like IV push tPA), you should be the one to make the call to the central pharmacy. Your familiarity with your department and colleagues will allow for faster dispensing of unconventional therapies in emergency scenarios.

Learn about the non-pharmacy equipment used in medical emergencies

At many emergencies there will be periods of time when the patient will not have any pharmacotherapy needs. When this happens you can still assist the team by being an extra pair of hands. Take the time to learn things like:

- What does an end tidal CO_2 detector look like?
- What drawer is an IV start kit kept in?
- Where is the on switch for the defibrillator?

If your hospital has a clinical nurse educator, seek them out. They will have access to a training version of a code cart and will be happy to go over it with you.

Expect some false alarms

Housekeeping might accidentally hit the code button. A patient might have fainted but is alert and talkative by the time the code team arrives. A floor nurse might call a rapid response on a patient that does not seem to have anything wrong.

Whatever the cause, it is important to never speak negatively about a 'false alarm' code or rapid response. If others overhear such talk, they may be hesitant to call for help again out of shame or embarrassment.

Think of the model that the cardiac catheterization lab employs to be on call 24/7 for STEMI patients. The team knows that once in awhile, the ECG will be misread. When the team is called in at 3am for a 'false alarm' they do not shame the ED physician / provider for not getting the call right; they know if they do, the same physician / provider might be hesitant to call the team in the future.

Chapter 2

Patient Assessment

You will encounter plenty of 'gray areas' for medication dosing when responding to medical emergencies. What if the patient's renal function is right on the cusp of a decision point for dose reduction? Should you really cut the antibiotic dose in half for a septic patient because their creatinine clearance is 49 instead of 51?

To help guide medication dosing in these 'gray areas,' you will want to make an assessment of how sick the patient is. Assessing how sick the patient is will help you prioritize the patient's problems and your response during the emergency.

Begin your assessment of how sick the patient is by deciding which of these two categories describes the patient's emergency:

1. A vital organ system *has failed* and it must be supported for the patient to survive.

2. Something has happened that indicates a vital organ system *might fail* in the near future.

Make patient focused risk:benefit assessments

When responding to medical emergencies, use your assessment of how sick the patient is to make patient focused risk:benefit assessments. Here are two examples that explain how deciding which category an emergency falls under can help with making patient focused risk:benefit assessments:

Example 1 - Opioid overdose

Imagine two different patients s/p hip fracture surgery that are experiencing effects from excessive opioid doses. The first patient is drowsy but opens her eyes if you call her name loudly. Her respiratory rate is 10 breaths per minute and her oxygen saturation is 92%. The second patient does not respond to voice or touch - only painful stimuli. Her respiratory rate is 6 breaths per minute and her oxygen saturation is 80%.

The first patient is showing signs that her respiratory system might fail if something is not done quickly. The second patient is showing signs that her respiratory system has failed and must be supported immediately in order to prevent cardiopulmonary arrest.

Both patients should receive naloxone for opioid overdose. The risk of causing opioid withdrawal with naloxone (and therefore extreme pain since the patients are s/p hip fracture surgery) versus the benefit of reversing the opioid effects is different in each patient. The first patient should be given a small dose of naloxone (0.04 to 0.08 mg) and be reassessed in 1 or 2 minutes to see if she starts to wake up. The second patient should be given a large dose of naloxone (at least 0.4 mg) and will need immediate airway management.

Example 2 - Massive pulmonary embolism

Imagine two different patients with massive pulmonary embolism. The first patient has a blood pressure of 85/55 mmHg, a heart rate of 55 beats per minute, and an oxygen saturation of 93%. The second patient has a blood pressure of 70/40 mmHg, a heart rate of 38 beats per minute, and an oxygen saturation of 85%.

Both patients should receive alteplase for the massive PE. The first patient should be given the standard IV infusion of 100 mg alteplase over 2 hours. The second patient's vital signs are much worse - cardiac arrest appears imminent. The second patient might not survive long enough for the 2 hour infusion of alteplase and therefore should be given IV push alteplase. Whatever risk may come with IV push alteplase is outweighed by the potential life saving benefit.

In the opioid overdose and pulmonary embolism examples, the difference between how sick the patients are may seem obvious. In reality the distinction may not be as clear. As you gain more experience responding to emergencies, you will become better at identifying how sick the patient is. If you are unsure, ask an experienced clinician their opinion. Critical care nurses in particular are excellent at assessing how sick a patient is.

Chapter 3

Verbal Communication

Effectively communicating your recommendation during an emergency is just as important as making the right recommendation in the first place.

Communication that occurs during medical emergencies is entirely verbal. The way the hospital system is setup, the physician / provider is the one person who can make the decision on what to order for a patient. To effectively communicate your recommendation, you will want to be able to talk like a physician and have the physician listen like a pharmacist. You can use a method called ISBAR to accomplish this:

Introduction (if the physician / provider does not know you)
Situation
Background
Assessment
Recommendation

Structuring your verbal communication using the ISBAR method helps you present your thoughts in a logical manner that allows the physician / provider to follow your decision-making process.

Let's use a patient example from Chapter 2, and apply the ISBAR method.

Take the opioid overdose patient who is s/p hip fracture surgery, drowsy but responds to voice, and has a respiratory rate of 10 breaths per minute and oxygen saturation of 92%. The physician / provider orders 0.4 mg naloxone IV push, but you think a lower dose should be used to avoid withdrawal since the patient's life is not threatened by the opioid effects. Here is how to communicate that using the ISBAR method:

Introduction: I'm Pharmacy Joe.
Situation: I'm concerned that 0.4 mg is more naloxone than the patient needs right now.
Background: She does not appear to be in respiratory failure and she's s/p hip fracture surgery.
Assessment: If we give 0.4 mg naloxone the patient may experience severe pain from opioid withdrawal.
Recommendation: Let's give a smaller dose like 0.08 mg of naloxone and wait a minute or two and see how she responds.

This recommendation can be presented in about 20 seconds and allows the physician / provider to understand the reasoning behind your recommendation.

In order to be able to present recommendations quickly using the ISBAR method, you will need to practice. A lot. This practice should occur outside of emergency situations in your day-to-day conversations with physicians / providers.

Earlier in my career I would literally sketch out the conversation before it happened using the ISBAR method. After doing that for a while, it has become second nature for me. Now I can use the ISBAR method to briefly and logically present a recommendation in any situation.

To help you practice using the ISBAR method, I have created a free tool that you can download at: pharmacyjoe.com/ISBARB

PART II

Chapter 4

Code Blue (Cardiac Arrest)

KEY POINTS

1. Follow ACLS protocols.

2. Assume responsibility for the provision of pharmacotherapy.

3. Actively participate in medical decision making to identify and reverse the cause(s) of the code.

4. Anticipate patient and provider needs and prepare in advance to meet those needs.

5. Function as a knowledgeable team member.

CODE BLUE TEAM PARTICIPATION

When pharmacists respond to code blue calls, patients die less often. A 2007 study associated pharmacist participation on cardiopulmonary resuscitation teams with 12,880 fewer deaths.

If a patient is to survive cardiopulmonary arrest, they need two things:

1. High quality uninterrupted chest compressions.
2. Rapid identification and correction of reversible causes. <--This is where a pharmacist can be most helpful.

Recommended certifications

Obtaining BLS and ACLS certifications are indispensable. Even if you never perform chest compressions during a code, BLS and ACLS certifications will be worthwhile. These certifications serve as a basic level of knowledge to make sure everyone is on the same page at the start of the code, minimize errors, and allow a team composed of strangers to be functional and successful.

ROLES AND EXPECTATIONS OF A PHARMACIST AT A CODE

Role 1 - Assume responsibility for the provision of pharmacotherapy:

- Locate and obtain necessary medications quickly and easily
- Calculate doses, rates, and concentrations correctly
- Prepare and label medications appropriately
- Provide IV compatibility information

Role 2 - Actively participate in medical decision making to identify and reverse the cause of the code:

- Make treatment recommendations
- Determine the cause of deterioration

Role 3 - Anticipate patient and provider needs and prepare in advance to meet those needs:

Always ask yourself "what is the worst thing that could go wrong right now?" Then obtain in advance the medications needed for the worst case scenario. *This is perhaps your most important role. If you have anticipated the patient's medication needs then you have greatly reduced the time from when the physician / provider decides a medication is needed to the time it is actually administered.*

Role 4 - Function as a knowledgeable team member:

- Make an effort to know the purpose and location of the non-medication contents of the code cart

Other team members you can expect at the code:

- Patient's nurse
- Critical care nurse
- Respiratory therapist
- Patient care technician
- Physician (hospitalist / intensivist / cardiologist / other)

HOW TO RESPOND TO THE CODE BLUE

Remain calm. Each code will be a different scenario; be alert and pay attention. You will become more confident after each code you attend. At my hospital, notification will come via the overhead page system and code beeper.

Get to work. If the medication tray has not been removed from the cart, remove it, place it on a flat surface, and open the plastic wrapping.

If the medication tray has already been removed, offer to assume responsibility for the medications.

Visually identify which team members are fulfilling the following roles:

- The physician / provider running the code
- The person recording events
- The nurse administering medications

Stand by the medication tray in sight of the physician / provider running the code.

If possible, be in view of the ECG monitor.

At the start of the code

At the start of the code open and assemble a 1 mg / 10 mL epinephrine syringe.

Obtain 6 normal saline flushes and prime them for use. To prime a saline flush: Remove the cap, slightly pull back on the plunger until you overcome the initial resistance, then push the plunger forward to remove air from the syringe and replace the cap. If the flush is not primed in this manner, the nurse may accidentally push too hard on the syringe to overcome the initial resistance; this could result in loss of the patient's IV access.

Assemble a few syringes and needles. Do this in advance to save time drawing up medications when they are requested later. I prefer to use 10 mL syringes. Locate additional supplies as necessary for requested medications. Stay focused on the physician / provider running the code.

Dispensing medications at a code

Loudly and clearly state the name and dose of the medication as you hand it over to the nurse.

Do not hand over an unlabeled medication! Pre-filled syringes are always pre-labeled, but anything you draw up in a syringe will need a label attached to it. Write the name and dose of the medication on a piece of 1 inch wide medical tape and then 'flag' the base of the syringe with this tape. If the medication is needed before you have time to write the label, tape the empty vial to the syringe as your 'label.' When you have a free moment, tear off a few strips of medical tape and pre-write labels for medications that you think might be requested.

Obtain or prepare another dose of the medication that was just used based on your knowledge of ACLS (i.e. epinephrine or amiodarone). This way you will have it ready to go when it is needed.

Keep track of empty boxes / vials, as the team often wants to know how many doses of the medications have already been used. Your recording nurse will thank you for this.

In conjunction with the recording nurse, keep track of the timing between doses of epinephrine. I use a timer on my smart watch (details at pharmacyjoe.com/smartwatchB) to do this - otherwise epinephrine will be requested far more frequently than ACLS protocols suggest.

Obtain patient allergies, weight, height, age, and gender from the medical record when time allows.

Always remain focused on the physician / provider running the code. In addition, be aware of events going on around you. An X-Ray technician may be waiting for you to step out of the room. Biohazardous products may be moving around you. A sterile field may have been set up that you need to steer clear of.

Obtain necessary medications that are not in the code cart by utilizing the appropriate resource; this may be a pharmacy technician outside the room or a phone call to the central pharmacy. Assist with post-resuscitation care if ROSC (return of spontaneous circulation) is obtained.

REFERENCES

Pharmacotherapy. 2007;27(4):481–493
Circulation. 2015;132(suppl 2):S315-589
Web-Based Integrated ACLS guidelines: eccguidelines.heart.org

Chapter 5

Rapid Response

KEY POINTS

1. Obtain needed medications.

2. Look for medication related causes of the patient's deterioration.

3. Assist the team as needed, often by reading aloud recent labs and medications administered.

4. Anticipate and prepare in advance for the patient's pharmacotherapy needs.

RAPID RESPONSE TEAM PARTICIPATION

A rapid response team (RRT) is a team of health care providers that responds to hospitalized patients with early signs of clinical deterioration on non-critical care units to prevent further deterioration to respiratory or cardiac arrest.

At my hospital anyone can call for the RRT, but it is usually the bedside nurse who makes the call.

RRT members:

- Critical Care Nurse
- Respiratory Therapist
- Hospitalist
- Pharmacist

RRT notification:

A beeper system is used at my hospital to notify the rapid response team.

Pharmacist's role:

- Obtain needed medications
- Look for medication related causes of the patient's deterioration
- Assist the team as needed, often by reading aloud recent labs and medications administered
- Anticipate and prepare in advance for the patient's pharmacotherapy needs

Problem identification:

Problems encountered during rapid response calls are primarily due to problems with oxygen delivery or ATP generation (hypoglycemia).

Oxygen Delivery = Stroke Volume x Heart Rate x Hemoglobin x

% Oxygen Saturation

At each rapid response call, focus on identifying the cause of decreased oxygen delivery.

CAUSES OF LOW % OXYGEN SATURATION

Functional airway obstruction:

Caused by a decreased level of consciousness whereby muscles relax and allow the tongue to obstruct the pharynx.

Treatments include:

- Airway maneuvers
- Antidote therapy
- Intubation

Mechanical airway obstruction:

This could be caused by aspiration of a foreign body, angioedema, bleeding, or stridor.

Treatments include:

- Anaphylaxis treatment
- Nebulized racemic epinephrine
- Intubation (likely will be difficult) or surgical airway

Remember the requirements for normal breathing:

- An intact respiratory center in the brain
- Intact nervous pathways from brain to diaphragm and accessory muscles
- Adequate diaphragm and accessory muscle function
- Unobstructed flow

Respiratory rate is an important indicator of inadequate oxygen delivery:

Lack of oxygen $\rightarrow$ anaerobic respiration $\rightarrow$ lactic acidosis $\rightarrow$ tachypnea

Other causes of low % oxygen saturation:

- Pulmonary embolism
- Shunting

CAUSES OF LOW HEMOGLOBIN

- Blood loss
- Coagulopathy
- Hemolysis (might be from medications!)
- Disseminated intravascular coagulation

CAUSES OF LOW CARDIAC OUTPUT

Cardiac output = stroke volume x heart rate

Decreased stroke volume which could be from:

- Decreased contractility
- Myocardial infarction
- Acidosis
- Medications

Decreased preload which could be from:

- Low intravascular volume (blood loss, sepsis)
- High intra-thoracic pressure (after intubation)

Fall in systemic vascular resistance which could be from:

- Sepsis, pancreatitis, decompensated liver disease
- Any medication that blocks the sympathetic nervous system (metoprolol, clonidine)

Other causes:

- Bradycardia
- Direct action on arteriole smooth muscle
- Medications
- Hyperthermia

LOOK FOR THE CONSEQUENCES OF HYPOTENSION

Inadequate CO → inadequate O2 delivery→ organ failure→ lactate formation → shock

Altered mental status and oliguria are two easy ways to look for organ failure.

CAUSES OF ALTERED MENTAL STATUS

- Decreased oxygen delivery
- Decrease blood glucose
- Medication toxicity - check pupils:
    Big pupils = sympathetic overactivity, anticholinergic toxicity
    Small pupils = opioid toxicity, cholinergic toxicity

MEDICATION TOXIDROMES

4 common medication toxidromes are:

- Anticholinergic
- Cholinergic
- Opioids
- Sympathomimetics

Toxidrome: Anticholinergic

Blood Pressure	-/↑
Pulse	↑
Respiratory Rate	±
Temperature	↑
Mental Status	Delirium
Pupil Size	↑
Peristalsis	↓
Diaphoresis	↓

Adapted From Goldfranks ↑ = increases ↓ = decreases ± = variable - = change unlikely

Toxidrome: Cholinergic

Blood Pressure	±
Pulse	±
Respiratory Rate	-/↑
Temperature	-
Mental Status	Normal to Depressed
Pupil Size	±
Peristalsis	↑
Diaphoresis	↑

Adapted From Goldfranks ↑ = increases ↓ = decreases ± = variable - = change unlikely

Toxidrome: Opiate/EtOH/Sedative

Blood Pressure	↓
Pulse	↓
Respiratory Rate	↓
Temperature	↓
Mental Status	Depressed
Pupil Size	↓(opiates) ±(others)
Peristalsis	↓
Diaphoresis	-

Adapted From Goldfranks ↑ = increases ↓ = decreases ± = variable - = change unlikely

Toxidrome: Sympathomimetics

Blood Pressure	↑
Pulse	↑
Respiratory Rate	↑
Temperature	↑
Mental Status	Agitated
Pupil Size	↑
Peristalsis	-/↑
Diaphoresis	↑

Adapted From Goldfranks ↑ = increases ↓ = decreases ± = variable - = change unlikely

27

REFERENCES

J Pharm Pract. 2016 Apr;29(2):116-20.
Goldfrank's Toxicologic Emergencies, 2015, 10e, McGraw-Hill
Pharmacists to the Early Rescue: http://www.ihi.org/resources/
Pages/ImprovementStories/PharmaciststotheEarlyRescue.aspx
COMPASS Training Manual: https://www.hse.ie/eng/about/Who/
clinical/natclinprog/acutemedicineprogramme/earlywarningscore/
compasstrainingmanual.pdf

Chapter 6

Shock

KEY POINTS

1. Obtain medications to facilitate endotracheal intubation (see page 55), IV fluids, and vasopressors (see page 35) to maintain circulation.

2. Further treatment depends on the etiology of shock:

- Tension pneumothorax or Pericardial tamponade? --> Obtain 1% lidocaine for injection to facilitate needle thoracostomy
- Massive pulmonary embolism? --> See page 73
- Dissection of the ascending aorta? --> Obtain IV morphine and labetalol or esmolol
- Hemorrhagic shock? --> Obtain sodium bicarbonate, calcium, and applicable anticoagulant reversal agents such as tranexamic acid, idarucizumab or 4-factor prothrombin complex concentrate
- Septic shock? --> See page 35
- Anaphylactic shock? --> See page 49

OBSERVATIONS

During the treatment of shock, the patient's life hangs in the balance while the care team quickly delivers interventions to identify and treat the underlying cause. Many of these interventions require medications to facilitate treatment.

I see the pharmacist's role in the treatment of shock as "setting the table" by having the necessary medications immediately available so the rest of the team can deliver supportive care or other interventions to the patient.

Recognizing shock

Typical features of shock include:

- Altered mental status
- Tachycardia
- Hypotension
- Oliguria
- Cool, clammy skin
- Metabolic acidosis

INTERVENTIONS

Supportive care

Airway, breathing, and circulation need to be addressed immediately. Obtain medications to facilitate endotracheal intubation, IV fluids, and vasopressors to maintain circulation. You might not have a central line at first but this is not a reason to delay the administration of vasopressors.

Any (IV) port in a storm.

Types of shock

Here are different types of shock states and the medications you will need at the bedside for treatment:

Anaphylactic shock

Anaphylactic shock occurs from an IgE-mediated allergic reaction to food, insect sting, or medication. The pharmacologic treatments for anaphylaxis are discussed in Chapter 8. The only medication that matters is epinephrine. It should be given IM 0.3 to 0.5 mg into the mid-outer thigh. If needed, this dose may be repeated every 5 to 15 minutes.

Tension pneumothorax

A tension pneumothorax is a build-up of air in the pleural space which obstructs venous return to the heart. Tension pneumothorax may occur after trauma, procedures, or mechanical ventilation. Treatment involves needle thoracostomy or the emergent placement of a chest tube to relieve the build-up of air. If the patient is awake and time allows, obtain 1% lidocaine for infiltration and local anesthesia.

Pericardial tamponade

Pericardial tamponade is caused by blood or fluid building up in the space between the myocardium and pericardial sac. Treatment involves emergent pericardiocentesis to drain the fluid. Sedation is rarely required. Obtain 1% lidocaine to anesthetize the puncture site and pericardium.

Hemorrhagic shock

Hemorrhagic shock may be traumatic or non-traumatic. Blood products and supportive care are the mainstays of treatment. Based on the history of present illness, reversal agents such as plasma, tranexamic acid, idarucizumab and 4-factor prothrombin complex concentrate may be called for. These agents reverse coagulopathies immediately but hemostasis will still take hours to achieve.

Aggressive supportive care is critical to give the patient time to achieve hemostasis. Additional therapies to correct metabolic derangements and promote hemostasis include sodium bicarbonate and calcium (also known as clotting factor IV).

Life-threatening tachyarrhythmia

Life-threatening tachyarrhythmias should be immediately cardioverted!!! For synchronized cardioversion in a shocked patient with a tachyarrhythmia use the minimum amount of sedation necessary. I prefer etomidate ~0.1mg/kg IV but low doses of midazolam may also be used. If the tachyarrhythmia is regular and narrow-complex, obtain adenosine as it may be requested by the physician / provider.

Life-threatening bradyarrhythmia

For life-threatening bradyarrhythmia, atropine will be the first treatment at a dose of 0.5 mg IV every 3 minutes to a max of 3mg. If this fails, transcutaneous pacing may be used. If the patient is awake, they will require sedation. I prefer to use IV benzodiazepines at the minimum dose necessary. IV infusions of dopamine (2-10 mcg/kg/min) or epinephrine (2-10 mcg/min) may also be called for.

Septic shock

The pharmacologic treatments for septic shock are discussed in Chapter 7. Be prepared to obtain IV fluids, antibiotics, and vasopressors.

Cardiogenic shock from myocardial infarction

Patients with cardiogenic shock from myocardial infarction need to get to the cardiac catheterization lab immediately. Obtain IV morphine and the antiplatelets & anticoagulants used in your local protocol.

Cardiogenic shock from acute aortic or mitral valve insufficiency

Cardiogenic shock from acute aortic or mitral valve insufficiency is a surgical emergency. Medical therapy might include nitroprusside and dobutamine infusion.

Dissection of the ascending aorta

Dissection of the ascending aorta is a surgical emergency. Obtain IV morphine for pain relief. Hemodynamic parameters must be lowered to minimize aortic wall stress. Obtain IV labetalol or esmolol to reduce the heart rate to less than 60 beats per minute and systolic blood pressure to 100-120 mmHg. If the blood pressure is not at goal, nitroprusside should be used next.

Severe pulmonary embolism

Provided there are no contraindications, IV thrombolytics should be used for a patient with shock due to severe pulmonary embolism.

Adrenal crisis

Patients with shock and a history of glucocorticoid deficiency or withdrawal may have adrenal crisis. Obtain 4 mg IV dexamethasone. Ensure that appropriate lab tests (serum cortisol, ACTH, aldosterone, chemistries) have been drawn before giving dexamethasone.

REFERENCES

Circulation. 2009 Jun 30;119(25):3232-41
Web-Based Integrated ACLS guidelines: eccguidelines.heart.org

Chapter 7

Sepsis

KEY POINTS

1. Prepare for intubation if the patient is experiencing respiratory compromise.

2. Give a rapid (over 20-30 minutes) IV bolus of normal saline 30 mL/kg.

3. Attempt to get blood cultures before giving antibiotics, but do not delay antibiotics more than 45 minutes.

4. Give appropriate broad spectrum antibiotic therapy, taking into consideration the source of infection. Consider using simultaneous infusions or IV push antibiotic administration.

5. Start norepinephrine for hypotension that persists after fluid bolus. Use a high dose and titrate down for patients that are in extremis.

OBSERVATIONS

The treatment of severe sepsis / septic shock involves antibiotics and supportive care.

Definitions:

Sepsis: Life-threatening organ dysfunction caused by a dysregulated host response to infection.

Septic shock: Sepsis with circulatory and cellular/metabolic abnormalities profound enough to substantially increase mortality.

Clinical criteria:

Sepsis: Suspected or documented infection plus an acute increase of ≥ 2 SOFA points (a proxy for organ dysfunction).

Septic shock: Sepsis plus vasopressor therapy needed to elevate MAP ≥ 65 mmHg plus lactate > 2 mmol/L (18 mg/dL) after adequate fluid resuscitation.

INTERVENTIONS

Airway and breathing

A patient with severe sepsis / septic shock might need stabilization of their airway and breathing with mechanical ventilation. Chapter 9 provides a review of the role and expectations of a pharmacist during endotracheal intubation.

IV Fluids

After the airway is secure, IV fluids are the most important intervention for a patient with severe sepsis / septic shock.

Septic shock is a distributive shock state. The intravascular volume is low, and therefore stroke volume and oxygen delivery are reduced. Giving IV fluids directly replenishes the intravascular volume, increases the stroke volume, and increases oxygen delivery.

Despite a lack of focus on IV fluids in my training, I have learned to treat them as a medication that requires a specific dose to be effective. The first thing to focus on when you encounter a patient with severe sepsis or septic shock is getting the right dose of IV fluid.

Nearly all patients with severe sepsis / septic shock will need a 30 mL/kg bolus or 2 or more liters of crystalloid IV fluid such as normal saline or lactated ringers.

This bolus of IV fluids will need to be administered over 20-30 minutes. Most IV pumps have a maximum rate of 999 mL/hour. Consult with the patient's nurse to determine if they think the patient's IV access is sufficient to get the bolus administered fast enough off the pump. If the IV pump turns out to be faster due to small IV lines, ask for 2 IV sites, each with a liter of IV fluid running at 999 mL/hour.

Nurses on general medical units may not be aware of or comfortable with the fast rate necessary to give an IV fluid bolus, and you will need to be assertive to get the IV fluids dosed correctly.

Vasopressors

Always obtain a bag of norepinephrine early on when encountering a patient with severe sepsis / septic shock. Although push-dose vasopressors are often advocated, the practice (beyond an occasional 1-time dose) is unnecessary if a pharmacist is present and able to facilitate starting an infusion.

Vasopressor Choice in Sepsis

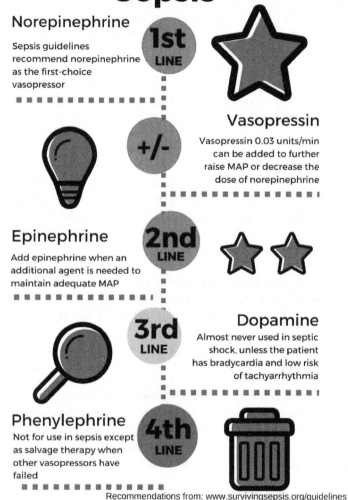

Norepinephrine

Sepsis guidelines recommend norepinephrine as the first-choice vasopressor

1st LINE

+/-

Vasopressin

Vasopressin 0.03 units/min can be added to further raise MAP or decrease the dose of norepinephrine

Epinephrine

Add epinephrine when an additional agent is needed to maintain adequate MAP

2nd LINE

Dopamine

3rd LINE

Almost never used in septic shock, unless the patient has bradycardia and low risk of tachyarrhythmia

Phenylephrine

Not for use in sepsis except as salvage therapy when other vasopressors have failed

4th LINE

Recommendations from: www.survivingsepsis.org/guidelines

To get a free color PDF of this chart go to pharmacyjoe.com/pressorchartB

Starting dose

The starting rate depends on how close the patient is to death. If they are in extremis, start at the maximum rate and titrate down. If they are stable, start at the bottom and work up.

Maximum dose

Maximum doses of vasopressors vary greatly between institutions. It is likely that your hospital has arbitrarily set a maximum dose for each vasopressor.

Do not get too concerned about what the maximum dose is, as long as there is agreement across disciplines (intensivists, cardiologists, anesthesiologists). Maximum doses were invented to be exceeded, so do not be shocked when the physician /provider squeezes the IV bag of dopamine in while trying to stabilize a young overdose patient long enough for ECMO to be started.

Peripheral versus central line

Any (IV) port in a storm.

Many patients would suffer organ damage from profound hypotension if you waited for central line placement before administering vasopressors.

If you are using vasopressors in a peripheral line, you should choose a small bore in the largest vein possible. If the need for vasopressors persists, a central line should be placed as soon as possible.

In a Cochrane review, the average infusion duration that resulted in complications was 55 hours. This is especially important given the phentolamine shortage. I would not count on phentolamine alternatives (terbutaline and topical nitro paste) if I were you.

Norepinephrine

If you were going to choose one vasopressor to start first in a patient with shock, norepinephrine would be the one to choose. Sepsis guidelines say to use this first, and there is data suggesting lower mortality with norepinephrine versus dopamine in cardiogenic shock.

Norepinephrine is a potent α-adrenergic agonist with less pronounced β-adrenergic agonist effects. It causes vasoconstriction and to a lesser extent increases cardiac output and stroke volume.

Reported dose ranges for norepinephrine are 0.01 to 3.3 mcg/kg/minute. My hospital's maximum is 0.6 mcg/kg/min and starting concentration is 8 mg in 250 mL normal saline.

Vasopressin

Vasopressin is an endogenously secreted hormone. It constricts vascular smooth muscle directly via V1 receptors and also increases responsiveness of the vasculature to catecholamines.

In septic shock, endogenous supplies are quickly depleted, and patients are often exquisitely sensitive to 'vasopressin replacement therapy' at a dose of 0.03 or 0.04 units/minute. Sepsis guidelines recommend adding vasopressin to norepinephrine. This combination usually allows for a lower dose of norepinephrine to be used.

Do not be surprised to see cardiac surgeons using vasopressin at higher doses for low cardiac output postoperatively. At my hospital, we use vasopressin up to 0.1 units/minute and titrate to effect (as opposed to fixed dosing in sepsis).

Epinephrine

Epinephrine is a more even mix of α and β agonist activity compared to norepinephrine.

It is reasonable to use epinephrine second line when other therapies are not enough.

Epinephrine causes more tachycardia and lactic acidosis than first line agents, and it should be weaned off first due to the risk of gut ischemia.

My hospital's starting concentration is 8 mg in 250 mL normal saline and maximum dose is 1 mcg/kg/minute.

Phenylephrine

You do not want to use this vasopressor if you do not have to, unless there is something benign going on like systemic vasodilation from medication effect (propofol) or epidural anesthesia. *The problem with phenylephrine is that it reduces cardiac output and decreases venous return.*

Phenylephrine is a pure α agonist. My hospital's starting concentration is 50 mg in 250 mL normal saline and maximum dose is 5 mcg/kg/minute.

DO NOT BE FOOLED into thinking that phenylephrine is first line in tachycardic patients because it has no β activity! Your shocked patient's tachycardia is probably a compensatory mechanism and will resolve after the shock is appropriately addressed.

Dopamine

Dopamine is like having 3 pressors in 1. Depending on the dose you can get dopamine to do a whole host of things.

Dopamine's activity is traditionally split into 3 categories with specific dose ranges, but in the critically ill patient there is often overlap between these categories:

1. < 5mcg/kg/minute - vasodilation in renal and mesenteric bed via dopaminergic receptors
2. 5-10 mcg/kg/minute - increased heart rate and contractility via β1 receptors
3. >10 mcg/kg/minute - arterial vasoconstriction via α1 receptors

It is important to know that dopamine has essentially no benefit over other vasopressors and comes with a higher risk of ventricular arrhythmia. Do not expect to use it much.

The starting concentration is 400 mg in 250 mL normal saline and my hospital's maximum rate is 20 mcg/kg/minute.

The one advantage dopamine does have is that it comes premixed with extended stability. This means you will more likely find it in a code cart.

You go to the code with the vasopressors you have, not the vasopressors you want to have.

Blood cultures before antibiotics (when possible)

You can blow your nose and clean your glasses with the same tissue, but you better do it in the right order.

Advocate for blood cultures prior to antibiotics, but do not withhold the antibiotics if it looks like blood cultures will not be readily obtained. Surviving Sepsis guidelines recommend no more than a 45 minute delay in antibiotics for the purpose of obtaining blood cultures first.

The rare case where you might run into a problem is giving antibiotics prior to cultures in a patient that turns out to have endocarditis. If their cultures come back negative because antibiotics were given first, they may need 6 weeks of broad spectrum therapy - yikes!

Antibiotics

If multiple antibiotics need to be given, run them simultaneously on different IV sites. The rare event of a patient reacting to an antibiotic and you not knowing which one, is outweighed by the delay that would occur in administering antibiotics sequentially.

Consider giving IV push antibiotics. If you can get your institution to adopt this practice, it will likely shorten the time it takes to give antibiotics to a septic patient. Most beta-lactam antibiotics are able to be given IV push.

Source identification and control

Source identification is generally taken care of by the physician / provider and it is very rare that I find myself adding to the care of the patient in this area. The easy things to look for are:

- Blood cultures
- Urinalysis (>20 WBC/HPF)
- Chest X-Ray (infiltrate)
- Physical exam (belly, skin wound, etc)

Antibiotics are not going to do much if source control is not obtained. Be aware of the patient management priority. Focus on what you can do to help ensure that source control can be achieved.

Antibiotic selection

Whenever possible look for a bacteriocidal antibiotic to give first as empiric therapy. Often this means choosing a beta-lactam antibiotic.

You need a 'cillin to do the killin'.

To help understand which antibiotics cover which type of pathogens, I have created a free visual critical care antibiotic guide. You can download it at: pharmacyjoe.com/abxguide

Lung

Community infection - ceftriaxone plus azithromycin or levofloxacin/moxifloxacin

Hospital infection - vancomycin plus piperacillin-tazobactam or cefepime

Aspiration - may consider adding anaerobic coverage (evidence is weak)

Brain

Community infection - the likely pathogens differ by age group - vancomycin, ceftriaxone, + ampicillin if over 50 years of age

Hospital or immune compromise - vancomycin, cefepime, and ampicillin

Necrotizing fasciitis

This is a surgical emergency! Do not do anything that will delay the patient's transportation to the operating room.

Pathogens include group A strep, anaerobes, MRSA, and the occasional gram negative - use linezolid + piperacillin / tazobactam or vancomycin + piperacillin / tazobactam + clindamycin

Clindamycin or linezolid should be part of every regimen until group A strep is ruled out. The purpose of these antibiotics is to shut down toxin production; they cannot be used alone due to being bacteriostatic.

Belly

You will need to cover gram negatives as well as anaerobes - use piperacillin / tazobactam or meropenem / imipenem / doripenem. A community acquired abdominal infection should not need empiric antifungal therapy. Nosocomial infections might need empiric antifungal therapy. If a critically ill patient has candida isolated, use micafungin until sensitivity data proves that fluconazole will be effective.

Unknown source

Use vancomycin + piperacillin / tazobactam or cefepime or meropenem. The sicker the patient, the broader the coverage should be.

Combination therapy versus pseudomonas aeruginosa

Your local resistance patterns dictate whether combination therapy against pseudomonas is necessary. Surviving Sepsis guidelines recommend (level 2B recommendation) empiric double coverage against pseudomonas in neutropenic patients for 3 to 5 days unless treatment can be narrowed sooner.

Renal dose adjustment of empiric antibiotic therapy

There are two reasons to adjust a medication for renal insufficiency: To prevent toxicity or to save money. My view is that there will be plenty of opportunity to reduce medication costs if the patient survives. If I am using a relatively non-toxic antibiotic (think anything with a beta-lactam ring) I will dose as per the patient's baseline renal function for the first 24 hours and then re-assess the dose.

Remember the serum creatinine lags actual improvement in kidney function and Cockcroft-Gault studied mostly 50 and 60 year olds who all had stable renal function.

COMPLICATIONS

Source control

Many patients with severe sepsis / septic shock will have an identifiable, focal source of the infection. This could range from an abscess that needs drainage to necrotizing fasciitis. While source control is out of the scope of a pharmacist, it is such an important part of the treatment of severe sepsis / septic shock. Keep these two things in mind regarding source control:

1. Do anything you can to facilitate source control. This might mean something as simple as holding the elevator open to get the patient to the operating room.

2. Do not do anything to delay source control. If a patient has necrotizing fasciitis, do not delay the patient's transport to the operating room even if the antibiotics have not been started yet. Instead make sure that anesthesia is aware and has the antibiotics in hand when the patient arrives in the pre-op area.

Is the patient responding?

During the treatment of a patient with severe sepsis / septic shock, keep an eye on signs of end-organ perfusion to help determine whether the patient is responding to the team's efforts.

Appropriate mental status, lactate clearance, urine output of 0.5mL/kg/hour or greater, and a mean arterial pressure of at least 65 mmHg are all excellent and minimally invasive ways of checking to see if the patient is responding to therapy.

REFERENCES

Trick of the Trade: IV-Push Antibiotics in the ED: https://www.aliem.com/2015/trick-iv-push-antibiotics/

Surviving Sepsis guidelines: http://www.sccm.org/Documents/
SSC-Guidelines.pdf
Specifications Manual for National Hospital Inpatient Quality
Measures, Version 5.0a
Am J Respir Crit Care Med. 2011 Apr 1;183(7):847-55.
Am J Respir Crit Care Med. Vol 171. pp 388–416, 2005.
Clin Infect Dis. 2007; 44:S27–72.
Clin Infect Dis. 2004; 39:1267–84.
Clin Infect Dis. 2010; 50:133–64.
Clin Infect Dis. 2014 Jul 15;59(2):147-59.

Chapter 8

Anaphylaxis

KEY POINTS

1. Epinephrine, IV fluids, and airway management are the main treatments for anaphylaxis.

2. Give epinephrine (1 mg per mL) 0.3 to 0.5 mg, injected IM into the mid-outer thigh. Repeat every 5 to 15 minutes if needed.

3. Do not delay giving epinephrine if anaphylaxis is suspected.

4. Steroids and antihistamines are not adequate to treat anaphylaxis and should not be given before or in place of epinephrine.

5. If the patient is beta-blocked give glucagon 1 to 5 mg IV over five minutes followed by an infusion of 5 to 15 mcg/minute.

OBSERVATIONS

A patient with anaphylaxis will often experience respiratory compromise, hypotension, and swollen lips-tongue-uvula.

Anaphylaxis is a potentially fatal allergic reaction with a rapid onset.

Immunoglobulin E (IgE) mediated allergic reactions to food, insect stings, and medications are the most common triggers for anaphylaxis.

As a result of the IgE reaction, mast cells release histamine and other mediators of anaphylaxis. If not properly treated, anaphylaxis will progress to respiratory arrest and cardiovascular collapse.

According to World Allergy Organization guidelines, anaphylaxis is highly likely when any one of the following three criteria is fulfilled:

1. Acute onset of an illness (within minutes to several hours) with involvement of the skin, mucosal tissue, or both (eg, generalized urticaria, itching or flushing, swollen lips-tongue-uvula)
AND AT LEAST ONE OF THE FOLLOWING:
A) Respiratory compromise (eg, dyspnea, wheeze-bronchospasm, stridor, reduced PEF, hypoxemia)
B) Reduced blood pressure or associated symptoms of end-organ dysfunction (eg. hypotonia [collapse], syncope, incontinence)

2. Two or more of the following that occur rapidly after exposure to a likely allergen for that patient (within minutes to several hours)
A) Involvement of the skin-mucosal tissue (eg, generalized

urticaria, itch-flush, swollen lips-tongue-uvula)
B) Respiratory compromise (eg, dyspnea, wheeze-
bronchospasm, stridor, reduced PEF, hypoxemia)
C) Reduced blood pressure or associated symptoms (eg,
hypotonia [collapse], syncope, incontinence)
D) Persistent gastrointestinal symptoms (eg, crampy
abdominal pain, vomiting)

3. Reduced blood pressure after exposure to known allergen
for that patient (within minutes to several hours)
A) Infants and children: low systolic blood pressure (age-
specific) or greater than 30% decrease in systolic blood
pressure
B) Adults: systolic blood pressure of less than 90 mm Hg or
greater than 30% decrease from that person's baseline

INTERVENTIONS

Epinephrine, IV fluids, and airway management are the main
treatments for anaphylaxis.

Epinephrine

Epinephrine is the medication of choice for anaphylaxis.
Epinephrine has no absolute contraindications to use in the
treatment of anaphylaxis.

Epinephrine stabilizes mast cells, prevents or reverses obstruction
to airflow in the upper and lower respiratory tracts, and prevents or
reverses cardiovascular collapse.

Intramuscular (IM) injection is the preferred route of
administration for the treatment of anaphylaxis. Several different
preparations of epinephrine are available - take care to select the
correct one! The epinephrine preparation for intramuscular

51

injection contains 1 mg per mL and will also be labeled as epinephrine 1:1000.

The recommended adult dose of epinephrine (1 mg per mL) is 0.3 to 0.5 mg per single dose, injected IM into the mid-outer thigh. If needed, this dose may be repeated every 5 to 15 minutes.

Occasionally, patients with extreme anaphylactic reactions do not adequately perfuse muscle tissue and therefore do not respond well to IM injection of epinephrine. If this occurs, administer epinephrine via an infusion pump at a rate of 2 to 10 mcg/minute (or 0.1 mcg/kg/minute).

Glucagon

For patients who are receiving beta-blockers, epinephrine's effectiveness will be blunted, and hypotension and bradycardia may persist despite administration of epinephrine.

If this occurs, glucagon is an attractive option due to it's inotropic and chronotropic effects that are not mediated through beta-receptors. A dose of 1 to 5 mg in adults given IV over five minutes followed by an infusion of 5 to 15 micrograms per minute is recommended. Overly rapid administration of glucagon will induce emesis.

Adjunctive treatment

Treatment of anaphylaxis with medications other than epinephrine is not supported by evidence.

Rationale for adjunctive treatments are extrapolated from other disease states such as urticaria or asthma. The following four adjunctive treatments are commonly used despite lack of evidence for their benefit:

1. H1 antihistamines

H1 antihistamines such as diphenhydramine or cetirizine relieve itching and urticaria. They have no effect on any of the life-threatening symptoms of anaphylaxis.

2. H2 antihistamines

H2 antihistamines such as famotidine or ranitidine may provide some additional relief of hives. They have no effect on any of the life-threatening symptoms of anaphylaxis.

3. Glucocorticoids

Glucocorticoids have an onset of action that is measured in hours and are therefore not helpful in the acute treatment of anaphylaxis. They have been routinely given to patients with anaphylaxis with the hope of preventing biphasic, late phase, or protracted anaphylaxis but evidence of effect is lacking.

4. Bronchodilators

Albuterol may be used to treat bronchospasm that persists despite administration of epinephrine. Remember that mucosal edema is not reversed by albuterol. Only the alpha-1 adrenergic effects of epinephrine will do this.

COMPLICATIONS

Medication disease interactions

Medications may interact with the disease state of anaphylaxis.

Angiotensin converting enzyme (ACE) inhibitors

Angiotensin II production is a normal compensatory response to anaphylaxis. Expect patients who develop anaphylaxis while on ACE inhibitors to have particularly profound hypotension.

Beta-blockers

Beta-adrenergic blockers may make anaphylaxis more resistant to treatment by blocking the bronchodilator and cardiovascular effects of epinephrine. Glucagon is recommended in this scenario.

Pitfalls in anaphylaxis treatment

The successful treatment of anaphylaxis revolves around timely administration of an adequate dose of epinephrine. Here are three pitfalls to watch out for:

1. Any delay in administration of epinephrine.
2. Thinking that medications other than epinephrine are adequate to treat anaphylaxis.
3. Errors in epinephrine administration due to multiple / confusing dosage forms.

REFERENCES

World Allergy Organization Journal. 2011, 4:13
Emerg Med J. 2005 Apr;22(4):272-3.
Ann Emerg Med. 2000 Nov;36(5):462-8.

Chapter 9

Endotracheal Intubation

KEY POINTS

1. For induction use etomidate 0.3mg/kg IV, propofol 1.5 mg/kg IV, or ketamine 1.5 mg/kg IV.

2. For paralysis use succinylcholine 1.5 mg/kg IV or rocuronium 1.2 mg/kg IV.

3. Do not give paralytics unless someone in the room can perform an emergency cricothyrotomy.

4. Stay aware of the duration of action of the sedatives and paralytics used to maintain the comfort of the patient.

5. Obtain appropriate sedation to use post intubation.

6. Be prepared for hypotension to occur after intubation and have a liter of normal saline and a vasopressor readily accessible.

INTERVENTIONS

The following scenarios will be covered in this chapter:

- Crash airway
- Rapid sequence intubation
- Delayed sequence intubation
- Difficult airway predicted
- Awake airway
- Failed airway

Treat these scenarios similar to code blue and rapid response calls and focus on:

- Identifying and predicting patient and provider needs
- Preparing in advance to meet those needs

Crash airway

A crash airway exists when the patient is in cardiac or respiratory arrest or is otherwise near death.

Endotracheal intubation is attempted without medications.

If the patient is not relaxed, a single dose of a paralytic (usually succinylcholine) may be given. Use 2mg/kg for this indication. This is a larger dose than usual but is given to ensure success.

Rapid sequence intubation (RSI)

RSI is established as the best way to ensure airway placement success in the absence of a difficult airway.

RSI is described as occurring in seven phases:

1. Preparation
2. Preoxygenation
3. Pretreatment

4. Paralysis with induction
5. Positioning
6. Placement
7. Post intubation

Preparation

While other clinicians are setting up supplies and equipment to perform the intubation, identify the medications that the physician / provider wants to use for paralysis and induction.

A general rule of thumb is to obtain double the amount of medication the physician / provider says they want. Nothing is worse than having to run to the medication room to get more induction agent after the procedure has started.

Preoxygenation

Preoxygenation is critical to maximize the 'safe apnea time' for the patient. This is the time the physician / provider has to place the airway after the patient stops breathing and before their O2 saturation drops to dangerous levels. Safe apnea time may be 8 minutes for a healthy adult, or less than 4 minutes for a critically ill or obese adult.

In this phase there is not much for the pharmacist to do, so continue with preparing / labeling if needed. If you have time, lay several blank pieces of tape out on a table so that you have labels ready to go if additional medications are called for.

Pretreatment

In the ICU I rarely use these pretreatment methods but I included them here as they are sometimes used in the emergency department.

Pretreatment involves giving lidocaine and or fentanyl to prevent known complications of intubation in at risk patients. There are three main reasons to use pretreatment:

1. Reactive airway disease

Give lidocaine 1.5mg/kg IV to prevent bronchospasm.

2. Elevated intracranial pressure (ICP)

Give lidocaine 1.5mg/kg IV to mitigate increased ICP from airway manipulation AND fentanyl 3mcg/kg IV to mitigate catecholamine surge from pain due to intubation.

3. Cardiovascular or other conditions when an acute rise in blood pressure or heart rate must be avoided

Give fentanyl 3mcg/kg IV to mitigate catecholamine surge from pain due to intubation.

Paralyze plus induction

This is supposed to occur simultaneously, but usually is given sequentially through the same IV line.

Give induction medication first in case something happens to the IV line.

Paralytics

There are 2 realistic options:

1. Succinylcholine 1.5 mg/kg IV
2. Rocuronium 1.2 mg/kg IV

Whether to use succinylcholine or rocuronium has been the subject of endless debate in medical literature as well as online medical communities. I believe the differences between the two medications are marginal and largely academic. Whichever paralytic the physician / provider is most familiar with is the one that should be used.

Induction agents

There are three realistic options:

1. Propofol 1.5 mg/kg IV

Propofol is a good choice if the patient is not critically ill and has good cardiovascular reserve. Expect propofol to cause some hypotension / bradycardia, especially if the patient is critically ill.

2. Ketamine 1.5 mg/kg IV

Ketamine is a good choice to use if the patient is critically ill or hemodynamically unstable. Ketamine's sedative effects are either on or off; they do not exist in a continuum like other sedatives. For this reason, I never give less than 1.5 mg/kg IV when using ketamine for induction.

3. Etomidate 0.3 mg/kg IV

Using etomidate for induction is nearly always a good choice. Expect this to be hemodynamically neutral. Some providers think even one dose of etomidate can cause adrenal insufficiency but the authors of Rosen's Emergency Medicine as well as the Cochrane reviewers state that this is not likely a concern.

A quick note on dosing - no patient was ever hurt by rounding up the dose for any RSI medication. The consequences of too little medication far outweigh the consequences of too much in this scenario so do not be stingy with your dosing!

Position the patient for intubation

Paralyzing the patient before they are in position for intubation makes me nervous, but this is where the experts put it in the RSI algorithms.

Placement

During this phase watch and listen for patient or physician / provider needs such as an unexpected difficult airway, hemodynamic changes, or inadequate sedation or paralysis.

Post intubation management

While the rest of the team is confirming tube placement and gas exchange, the pharmacist should be focused on the continued sedation and comfort of the patient.

Obtaining continuous sedation infusions can be time consuming; ask for some midazolam (0.05mg/kg or more) and fentanyl (1mcg/kg or more) IV boluses to be given while the continuous sedation regimen is selected and obtained.

Hypotension often occurs following emergency intubation. Venous return is reduced by the positive pressure in the intrathoracic cavity that the ventilator induces. The initial treatment for this is a saline or lactated ringers bolus followed by a norepinephrine infusion if needed.

While 'push dose pressors' are tempting to use, I prefer continuous IV administration of vasopressors instead. The reason is that when using 'push dose pressors,' the physician / provider must remember to give them every few minutes. This effectively gives the most experienced person in the room a role that a machine (a smart pump) can perform. Vasopressor administration must occur immediately when it is needed so I always prepare ahead of time a liter of normal saline, a bag of norepinephrine, IV tubing, and 2 IV pumps.

Delayed sequence intubation (DSI)

DSI is proposed for use when the patient cannot tolerate preoxygenation (usually due to agitation).

DSI is essentially procedural sedation with 1.5mg/kg IV ketamine so that the patient can tolerate the 'procedure' of preoxygenation. RSI then proceeds when preoxygenation is complete. Ketamine is chosen because the patient will be sedated but maintain respirations with this medication.

A criticism of DSI is that it is not well studied and only has case series and case reports to support its use. DSI is about as well studied as parachute use to prevent death and major trauma from gravitational challenge. I will take the parachute any time!

Difficult airway predicted

Predicting a difficult airway is not necessary for a pharmacist, but knowledge of how to do so can be obtained by reviewing the chapter in Rosen's Emergency Medicine on Airway Management, or any number of other resources.

In this setting the patient may be sedated more like procedural sedation without the use of paralytics. Induction agents may be titrated and the patient may only reach a moderate / deep level of sedation.

A glidescope is always used for difficult airways at my hospital.

A majority of the airways placed in my medical / surgical community ICU appear to fall under this category with paralytics being withheld and sedatives being titrated.

Awake airway

I can only remember an awake fiberoptic intubation once in an obese patient with myasthenia crisis. After several failed attempts, we administered a 1mcg/kg IV bolus over 10 minutes of dexmedetomidine and the patient was successfully intubated.

Failed airway

A failed airway exists when further attempts at endotracheal intubation are unlikely to result in an airway being placed. A laryngeal mask airway or cricothyrotomy may be attempted in this case.

Other than possibly obtaining local anesthetic for use in the cricothyrotomy, the role of the pharmacist in this scenario is to make preparations to treat the patient should they progress to cardiac arrest.

Mechanical ventilation

Once the patient has been intubated they will be placed on mechanical ventilation. While pharmacists' knowledge of mechanical ventilation is outside the scope of this book, I have made available for free a 2 page PDF of what a pharmacist should know about mechanical ventilation at: pharmacyjoe.com/ventilationB

REFERENCES

Ann Emerg Med. 2005 Oct;46(4):328-36.
Ann Emerg Med. 2012 Mar;59(3):165-75.
Rosen's Emergency Medicine, 8e
Cochrane Database of Systematic Reviews 2015, Issue 1. Art. No.: CD010225.
Annals of Emergency Medicine. 2015, Apr;65(4):349 - 355.

Chapter 10

Stridor

KEY POINTS

1. Bring 2 ampules of racemic epinephrine (2.25%, 0.5 mL) and 8 mg IV dexamethasone to the bedside immediately.

2. Observe the patient, including their mental status and vital signs. If the patient with stridor is drowsy, immediately prepare for intubation.

3. Bring medications to support endotracheal intubation to the bedside:

- For induction use etomidate 0.3mg/kg IV, propofol 1.5 mg/kg IV, or ketamine 1.5 mg/kg IV.
- For paralysis use succinylcholine 1.5 mg/kg IV or rocuronium 1.2 mg/kg IV.

OBSERVATIONS

Stridor requires immediate attention. It is an abnormal inspiratory sound that represents upper airway obstruction.

Recognition

Stridor can be heard without a stethoscope. It is usually a high pitch sound that occurs during the inspiratory phase. Observe the patient from the end of the bed and see if the noise is worse when their chest expands (inspiration) or falls (expiration). A noise on inspiration is consistent with stridor. A noise on expiration indicates lower airway obstruction such as bronchospasm.

Causes

Stridor can be caused by a mass or foreign body in the upper airway, or by laryngeal edema. Laryngeal edema post endotracheal extubation is the most likely cause of stridor in an adult patient in the ICU.

INTERVENTIONS

Stridor is a sign of impending respiratory failure. If you hear a stridorous patient, or hear other clinicians saying that a patient has stridor, make the following three preparations:

1. Bring 2 ampules of racemic epinephrine (2.25%, 0.5 mL) and 8 mg IV dexamethasone to the bedside immediately.
2. Observe the patient, including their mental status and vital signs. If the patient with stridor is drowsy, intubation will be immediately necessary.
3. Bring medications to support endotracheal intubation to the bedside (covered in Chapter 9).

Racemic epinephrine via nebulization

Epinephrine causes vasoconstriction and decreased blood flow, which diminishes edema formation. Randomized controlled trials that prove efficacy of epinephrine in post-extubation laryngeal edema in adults are lacking.

There is no consensus about the potentially effective dosage of epinephrine nebulization. Rebound edema is known to occur and the patient should be monitored for this. At my hospital, the respiratory therapists like to repeat a dose of nebulized epinephrine. I make sure that two ampules of 2.25%, 0.5 mL racemic epinephrine are available.

Dexamethasone

Corticosteroids reduce edema by down-regulating inflammatory response and decreasing capillary vessel dilatation and permeability. The most effective dose has not been determined. I use 8 mg of dexamethasone based on prescribing patterns at my hospital.

Heliox

Helium administration can also be considered for stridor. Explaining heliox to my pharmacy students is a great way to illustrate how many therapies can be boiled down to simple high school level science.

Air is approximately 20% oxygen and 80% nitrogen. Replacing the nitrogen with helium results in a lower density gas. Because stridor is caused by turbulence in the airway, using a lower density gas causes less turbulence and therefore is beneficial in stridor. At my hospital our standard concentration for heliox is 30% oxygen and 70% helium. Evidence of its usefulness in adults with laryngeal edema is limited to case reports and nonrandomized trials.

REFERENCES

Hear what stridor sounds like: http://respwiki.com/ Breath_sounds#Stridor

J Intensive Care Med. 2004 Nov-Dec;19(6):335-44.

Rev Esp Anestesiol Reanim. 2009 May;56(5):319-21.

Cochrane Database Syst Rev. 2006 Oct 18;(4):CD002884.

Crit Care. 2015; 19(1): 295.

Chapter 11

Methemoglobinemia

KEY POINTS

1. Suspect methemoglobinemia when the following occur:

- Sudden cyanosis after ingestion of a medication that may cause methemoglobinemia
- Hypoxia that does not improve with increasing amounts of oxygen
- Chocolate brown or otherwise discolored blood during phlebotomy

2. Immediately obtain methylene blue and give 1 to 2 mg/kg IV over 5 minutes if the methemoglobin levels are 20% or higher or the patient is symptomatic.

OBSERVATIONS

There are two types of methemoglobinemia; congenital and acquired. This chapter covers the recognition and treatment of acquired methemoglobinemia.

Background

Methemoglobin is formed when the ferrous irons of heme are oxidized to the ferric state. The ferric hemes of methemoglobin are unable to bind oxygen therefore causing a functional anemia.

Acquired methemoglobinemia is typically a reaction to medications. The most common medications that cause this reaction are benzocaine, prilocaine, lidocaine, and dapsone.

Several other medications and chemicals have been reported to cause methemoglobinemia: Chloroquine, ammonium nitrate, nitrous oxide, phenytoin, metoclopramide, anilines, automobile exhaust fumes, toluidine, primaquine, silver nitrate, sulfamethoxazole, valproate, butyl nitrite, benzene, oral hypoglycemics, chlorates, sodium nitrate, nitroglycerine, sulfadiazine, flutamide, naphthalene, isobutyl nitrite, nitric oxide, nitroprusside, sulfones, nitrofurantoin, alloxan, and paraquat.

Recognition of acquired methemoglobinemia

The signs of methemoglobinemia depend on the degree of methemoglobin:

10-20% - cyanosis, blue or gray appearing skin, lips, and nail beds
20-30% - lightheadedness, anxiety, headache, tachycardia
30-50% - fatigue, confusion, dizziness, tachypnea
50-70% - coma, seizures, acidosis, arrhythmia
>70% - death

Pulse oximetry is inaccurate in the presence of significant methemoglobinemia and cannot be relied on.

Suspect methemoglobinemia when the following occur:

- Sudden cyanosis after ingestion of a medication that may cause methemoglobinemia
- Hypoxia that does not improve with increasing amounts of oxygen
- Chocolate brown or otherwise discolored blood during phlebotomy

Several years ago I encountered a 60 y/o male s/p transesophageal echocardiogram (TEE) who developed sudden cyanosis, tachycardia and confusion at the end of his procedure. Oxygen was applied, a rapid response was called, and a blood gas was drawn by a respiratory therapist. The therapist immediately noticed a chocolate brown discoloration of the patient's blood and suspected methemoglobinemia. We then discovered the patient had been given topical benzocaine spray prior to the TEE. As the blood gas was being tested in the lab I obtained methylene blue from the main pharmacy and started to determine what dose would be needed if the sample was positive for methemoglobin.

In our case, methemoglobinemia was suspected from the onset and so the first blood gas sample was checked for the % methemoglobin.

But what if you did not suspect methemoglobinemia until after the blood gas was drawn? Check to see if the pulse oximetry is 90% or less and the blood gas pO2 is 70 mmHg or higher; if it is, methemoglobinemia is suspected.

INTERVENTIONS

Methylene blue

Methylene blue accelerates the conversion of methemoglobin to hemoglobin, effectively reversing the functional anemia caused by methemoglobinemia. Because high levels of methemoglobinemia are a medical emergency, methylene blue should be obtained and brought to the bedside the moment methemoglobinemia is suspected.

Treatment with methylene blue should be given whenever the methemoglobin levels are 20% or higher or the patient is symptomatic. The patient should be transferred to an ICU setting so that the patient's respiratory and cardiovascular systems can be supported if needed. Paradoxically, at high doses, methylene blue can actually cause methemoglobinemia.

Dosing

1 to 2 mg/kg IV over 5 minutes of methylene blue should be given immediately if the methemoglobin levels are 20% or higher or if the patient is symptomatic. The dose can be repeated in 1 hour if needed.

The administration of methylene blue will render standard detection of methemoglobin inaccurate, and other methods must be used.

Most patients will improve rapidly and not require any further treatment.

Contraindications and monitoring

Methylene blue is contraindicated in G6PD deficiency, although pre-treatment screening for this is impractical.

Methylene blue rarely causes serotonin syndrome.

Alternative treatments

Intravenous ascorbic acid has been used when methylene blue is unavailable. Blood transfusions may be considered as well, depending on the severity of disease.

REFERENCES

Indian J Crit Care Med. 2014 Apr; 18(4): 253–255.
SQU Med J, May 2012, Vol. 12, Iss. 2, pp. 237-241, Epub. 9th Apr 2012
Anesth Analg. 2009 Mar;108(3):837-45.
J. Biol. Chem. 1938 126: 655

Chapter 12

Massive Pulmonary Embolism

KEY POINTS

Obtain 100 mg alteplase if the patient has an acute pulmonary embolism (PE) and any of the following:

- Hypotension
- Profound bradycardia (<40 beats per minute)
- Cardiac arrest

OBSERVATIONS

Massive pulmonary embolism (PE) is present when a patient has an acute PE and hypotension, profound bradycardia, or cardiac arrest.

When to give alteplase

There is broad agreement among experts to administer alteplase in the setting of massive PE. It makes good sense considering the pathophysiology - the clot has to go for oxygenation to return. Anti-thrombotics like heparin and enoxaparin are not going to do a thing to the existing clot; they will just prevent the clot from getting bigger.

CHEST guidelines state: In patients with acute PE associated with hypotension (systolic BP , 90 mm Hg) who do not have a high bleeding risk, we suggest systemically administered thrombolytic therapy over no such therapy (Grade 2C) .

Why is alteplase given in massive PE

The hope is that mortality will be decreased by lysing the clot. In the 2012 CHEST guidelines, the authors note that there is only a trend pointing towards a mortality benefit with lytic therapy.

Since the publication of the CHEST guidelines there has been a meta-analysis which points to an association with lower all-cause mortality with lytic therapy. However the wide range of patient groups and treatments in this meta-analysis leaves many unanswered questions.

Even though the available evidence is less than ideal, I doubt further trials will compare lytic therapy to placebo in massive PE given the clear pathophysiology and rationale for lytics. As the CHEST guidelines state: Patients with the most severe presentations who have the highest risk of dying from an acute PE have the most to gain from thrombolysis.

Plenty of 'soft endpoints' are improved after alteplase is given for massive PE. Clot lysis is accelerated and there is early hemodynamic improvement (eg, improved pulmonary arterial blood pressure, right ventricular function, and pulmonary perfusion). There is, as you would expect, an increased risk of major bleeding.

In most cases, thrombolytic therapy should be considered only after acute PE has been confirmed because the bleeding events after thrombolytic therapy can be severe.

INTERVENTIONS

How to give alteplase for massive PE

There are three options for alteplase administration in massive PE. They are catheter directed therapy, IV push, or IV infusion.

1. Catheter directed therapy

For massive PE, this is a fringe option and would only be used for patients who do not have a low bleeding risk but still appear to need lytic therapy. Catheter directed therapy involves infusing alteplase into the pulmonary artery at a rate of 0.5 to 2 mg/hour. An ultrasound device may be used to assist in the delivery of alteplase, with the ultrasound creating additional surface area on the clot for the alteplase to lyse.

Another role for catheter directed lytic therapy in massive PE is as a 'rescue' therapy if systemic thrombolysis has failed.

2. IV push

If a patient with an acute PE appears to have an imminent cardiac arrest, or has already arrested, alteplase should be given IV push. CHEST guidelines specifically state this, so you can be confident you are not out on a limb if this is being ordered. IV push alteplase is always a disturbing thought for pharmacists but remember the pathophysiology; if the clot does not go away, the patient will not get any oxygen. Data suggest that longer alteplase infusion times are associated with higher bleeding risk compared to shorter infusion times.

Case reports and series have reported some success from systemic thrombolytic therapy during cardiopulmonary resuscitation when the cardiac arrest is due to suspected or confirmed acute PE.

3. IV infusion

If the patient has a pulse and is of low bleeding risk, IV infusion is the way alteplase should be given. I typically use 100 mg IV over 2 hours but there have been additional studies suggesting that 50 mg IV over 15 minutes is just as safe and effective. The CHEST guidelines note that the 100 mg over 2 hours regimen has been studied more extensively.

Bleeding risk

Robust data on bleeding risk is lacking. The CHEST authors assume that the bleeding risk with thrombolytic therapy is similar in patients with PE as with acute ST-segment elevation myocardial infarction. This puts the risk of intracranial hemorrhage (ICH) at about 1% or less. Other serious types of bleeds are more common, but because the risk of ICH is so much lower than when alteplase is given for stroke, most clinicians I have talked to agree that patients who receive alteplase for PE do not need the same type of neurologic monitoring as those who receive it for stroke.

What to do with the heparin infusion

CHEST guidelines cover this very well. They say it is acceptable to either continue or suspend the UFH infusion during administration of thrombolytic therapy (these two practices have never been compared). During a 2 hour infusion of 100 mg of alteplase, US regulatory bodies recommend suspension of IV UFH, whereas IV UFH is continued during the alteplase infusion in many other countries. US authorities recommend checking the activated partial thromboplastin time immediately after completion of the alteplase infusion and, provided that the activated antithrombin time is not > 80 seconds, restarting IV UFH without a bolus at the same infusion rate as before alteplase was started.

Usually, after I inform the physician / provider of the statement in the CHEST guidelines they make the decision to hold the heparin infusion while the alteplase is running.

REFERENCES

Circulation. 2011 Apr 26;123(16):1788-830.
Chest. 2012;141(2_suppl):e419S-e494S.
JAMA. 2014 Jun 18;311(23):2414-21.
Crit Care Med. 2001 Nov;29(11):2211-9.
Arch Intern Med. 2000 May 22;160(10):1529-35.
Ther Adv Drug Saf. 2015 Apr; 6(2): 57–66.

Chapter 13

Status Epilepticus

KEY POINTS

1. Obtain lorazepam 0.1 mg/kg IV or midazolam 0.2 mg/kg IM.

2. Prepare to assist with supportive care.

3. Keep an eye on the clock with the goal of terminating seizure activity within 30 minutes.

OBSERVATIONS

Seizure

Whenever you encounter a hospital inpatient with an acute seizure, make sure that you have IV lorazepam available. Most seizures stop after about 2 minutes. In reality, this means that by the time the lorazepam has been brought to the bedside, the seizure is usually over.

When the seizure is over, assist the team in identifying and treating the underlying cause of the seizure. Common reasons for an adult inpatient to experience a seizure include:

- Intracerebral mass or bleed
- CNS infection
- Cerebral hypoxia
- Medication overdose (such as tricyclic antidepressants)
- Medication withdrawal (such as anticonvulsants, alcohol, or benzodiazepines)
- Metabolic disturbance (low glucose or sodium)

Status epilepticus

If the seizure lasts more than 5 minutes, the patient is now considered to be in status epilepticus.

Status epilepticus is a neurologic emergency and can result in respiratory failure, cardiovascular collapse, and neurologic damage if it is not terminated.

Rapid treatment is essential for a good patient outcome.

INTERVENTIONS

Guidelines for the treatment of status epilepticus published in 2012 are available from the Neurocritical Care Society.

Treatment should begin immediately with a benzodiazepine. Use lorazepam 0.1 mg/kg IV or midazolam 0.2 mg/kg IM.

Avoid giving midazolam IV because this is more likely to cause respiratory arrest and force endotracheal intubation upon a patient who might not have required it.

Immediately after benzodiazepines are given, obtain medications necessary to support the patient if they develop respiratory failure or hypotension. This involves preparing medications for endotracheal intubation (see Chapter 9) and vasopressor therapy (see Chapter 7).

Whether or not seizure activity has stopped after you have obtained intubation and vasopressor medications, an anti-epileptic medication will be needed. A 2014 article recommends levetiracetam (30 mg/kg IV), valproic acid (30 mg/kg IV), or phenytoin (20 mg/kg IV).

Refractory status epilepticus

Refractory status epilepticus is treated with general anesthesia and mechanical ventilation.

When status epilepticus is considered refractory is up for debate.

The 2012 guidelines state status epilepticus that persists after benzodiazepines and an anti-epileptic medication is considered refractory.

Some experts use an alternative definition of refractory status epilepticus. On an emcrit.org episode Tom Bleck stated: "Status epilepticus should be considered refractory after the failure of the first agent that should have worked."

The trouble with the guideline definition is that it assumes that an anti-epileptic medication is immediately available at the bedside to administer after initial benzodiazepines are given. In reality, ordering, preparing, dispensing and administering an IV anti-epileptic medication will take 20 minutes or more even in the most ideal circumstances.

In practice using the approach in the guidelines - waiting until an anti-epileptic medication fails to move to general anesthesia - may result in status epilepticus persisting for 60 minutes or more. The alternative definition of refractory status epilepticus serves to accelerate the time to general anesthesia and termination of status epilepticus. This is thought to be beneficial since the risk of serious neurologic damage increases greatly if seizure activity persists longer than 30 minutes.

At the time this book was published there is no study, either published or underway, that examines whether moving toward general anesthesia faster results in better outcomes.

General anesthesia regimens for terminating refractory status epilepticus

There are three options to consider for inducing anesthesia to terminate refractory status epilepticus:

1. Midazolam

Give 0.2 mg/kg IV followed by an infusion of at least 0.2 mg/kg/hour, titrating up to 2 mg/kg/hour. Watch out for tachyphylaxis which may necessitate dose increases.

2. Propofol

Give 2 mg/kg IV followed by an infusion of 50 mcg/kg/hour. Watch out for hypotension and give a vasopressor to counteract this.

3. Ketamine

Give 3 mg/kg IV followed by an infusion of at least 1 mg/kg/hour titrating up to 10 mg/kg/hour.

REFERENCES

Neurocrit Care. 2012 Aug;17(1):3-23.
Intensive Care Medicine. 2014 Sept;40(9):1359-1362.
Arch Neurol. 1973 Jan;28(1):10-7.

Chapter 14

Acute Agitation

KEY POINTS

1. Medication selection is based on the cause of agitation:

   - Unknown cause --> Use haloperidol 5 mg IM/IV plus lorazepam 2 mg IM/IV
   - Ethanol intoxication --> Use haloperidol 5 mg IM/IV
   - Medication intoxication or withdrawal --> Use lorazepam 2 mg IM/IV
   - Psychiatric disorder --> Use haloperidol 5 mg IM/IV

2. If excessive doses of benzodiazepines or antipsychotics are ineffective, ketamine may be used as a rescue treatment for acute agitation. The dose of ketamine is 2 mg/kg IV or 5 mg/kg IM.

OBSERVATIONS

Chemical sedation is part of the array of options to treat acute agitation. Prevention strategies, verbal de-escalation techniques, and physical restraints also play a role in the prevention and management of acute agitation.

The ideal first line medications to use for rapid tranquilization of an acutely agitated patient are benzodiazepines and antipsychotics. These medications may be given alone or in combination.

Evidence for the use of chemical sedation is limited to small trials of at most a few hundred patients. Midazolam and lorazepam are the most studied benzodiazepines and haloperidol and droperidol are the most studied antipsychotics. Generally, control of the patient's agitation is achieved within 15-20 minutes with these medications. The main side effect to monitor and be prepared for is respiratory depression.

INTERVENTIONS

Medication selection is based on cause of agitation:

Unknown cause

When the cause of acute agitation is unknown, use combination therapy with haloperidol 5 mg IM/IV and lorazepam 2 mg IM/IV. This combination works faster than using either medication alone. These two medications are compatible in syringe and should be mixed so that only one injection is needed.

Many providers at my hospital add 50 mg of diphenhydramine to the syringe, and call the combination a "B-52" for Benadryl + 5 mg haloperidol + 2 mg lorazepam. The sedating properties of antihistamines are well established, but this combination has never been studied to my knowledge.

Ethanol intoxication

When the cause of acute agitation is ethanol intoxication, use an antipsychotic such as haloperidol 5 mg IM/IV first. Benzodiazepines given to a patient with ethanol intoxication may be more likely to cause respiratory depression.

Medication intoxication or withdrawal

When the cause of acute agitation is medication intoxication or withdrawal, use a benzodiazepine such as lorazepam 2 mg IM/IV. Antipsychotics can increase the seizure risk when given to patients in alcohol or benzodiazepine withdrawal, and can worsen anticholinergic toxicity.

Psychiatric disorder

When the cause of acute agitation is a psychiatric disorder, use an antipsychotic such as haloperidol 5 mg IM/IV.

Frequent re-dosing of benzodiazepines or antipsychotics may be necessary to control agitation, and the interval between doses may need to be much shorter than the every 15 to 30 minutes that would otherwise be recommended for these medications. Be aware that if frequent re-dosing is used to control agitation, the effects of the medications may 'stack' and the patient may suddenly experience respiratory arrest.

I do not usually use the atypical antipsychotics in acute agitation, but they may be useful if the patient is semi-cooperative and willing to take an oral dissolving tablet such as olanzapine. Although the parenteral formulation of olanzapine is labeled for IM use only, some authors have published data suggesting that IV olanzapine may be used.

Ketamine if other medications are ineffective

If excessive doses of benzodiazepines or antipsychotics are

ineffective, ketamine may be used as a rescue treatment for acute agitation. Ketamine has been used to successfully manage acutely agitated and violent patients. The dose for this indication is 2mg/kg IV or 5mg/kg IM. In addition to not requiring intubation, ketamine does have the advantage of possible IM injection, which may be the only choice in some agitated patients.

REFERENCES

Am J Emerg Med. 1997 Jul;15(4):335-40.
Pharmacotherapy. 1998 Jan-Feb;18(1):57-62.
Int Clin Psychopharmacol. 2015 May;30(3):142-50.
Crit Care. 2011; 15(5): R257.

Chapter 15

Severe Alcohol Withdrawal

KEY POINTS

1. Give diazepam IV 5 to 10 mg every 5 to 10 minutes until the patient is appropriately sedated.

2. Avoid dexmedetomidine as monotherapy.

3. If dexmedetomidine is used, ensure the patient continues to receive benzodiazepines.

4. Consider thiamine 250 mg IV q24 hours for prophylaxis of Wernicke's Encephalopathy.

OBSERVATIONS

Symptoms of alcohol withdrawal are the result of an increase in autonomic activity and sympathetic outflow, as well as psychomotor agitation. Commonly this manifests as diaphoresis, nausea, vomiting, tremor, and anxiety.

Severe alcohol withdrawal may progress to seizures and/or delirium tremens.

INTERVENTIONS

The goal of treatment is to reduce the severity of symptoms and prevent progression to delirium tremens.

It is widely accepted that the best way to treat alcohol withdrawal in hospitalized patients is with symptom-triggered benzodiazepine therapy. Such treatment results in equivalent outcomes and less benzodiazepine use compared with scheduled benzodiazepine therapy.

The use of symptom-triggered therapy has yet to be studied prospectively in patients requiring intensive care for severe alcohol withdrawal.

Evidence for treating severe alcohol withdrawal is limited to retrospective pre / post intervention reviews. From the available evidence, it appears that escalating doses of diazepam up to 100 mg per dose or more is a reasonable approach.

Diazepam

Diazepam is an ideal benzodiazepine to use for severe alcohol withdrawal. It is available in IV and oral form and has active metabolites which might provide longer duration of action and smoother clinical course.

The need for mechanical ventilation was reduced in two studies when protocol-based escalating doses of diazepam were used. One of the studies found a trend in decreased ICU length of stay while the other found a significant decrease from 9.6 to 5.2 days using protocol-based escalating doses of diazepam. The protocol-based escalating doses of diazepam for severe alcohol withdrawal were dosed to a target RASS goal of 0 to -2. The diazepam dose increased every 10 minutes up to 100-150 mg per dose. If agitation was not controlled at these doses, phenobarbital was added. If this did not work, continuous sedation and mechanical ventilation were employed.

It is counter-intuitive that high doses of benzodiazepines might prevent mechanical ventilation, but that is what the evidence suggests.

Give diazepam IV 5 to 10 mg every 5 to 10 minutes until the patient is appropriately sedated.

Dexmedetomidine

As an alpha-2 agonist, dexmedetomidine reduces sympathetic outflow and blunts many of the symptoms of alcohol withdrawal. Dexmedetomidine is not appropriate for monotherapy in severe alcohol withdrawal as it lacks the GABA receptor activity required to prevent seizures.

Many clinicians perceive that dexmedetomidine has the potential to spare the need for intubation in severe alcohol withdrawal. So far evidence only demonstrates that dexmedetomidine has the potential to reduce the use of benzodiazepines. Whether this translates to a decrease in length of stay or mortality is yet to be seen.

In my own practice I find that dexmedetomidine is frequently added too soon to patients with severe alcohol withdrawal. Often this is done before significant doses of benzodiazepines have been used.

Adding dexmedetomidine complicates the assessment of the symptoms of alcohol withdrawal. If only 'as needed' doses of benzodiazepines are ordered, dexmedetomidine often ends up being used as monotherapy. This leaves the patient at risk of alcohol withdrawal seizures. Anecdotally, I find these patients also have prolonged alcohol withdrawal symptoms.

If dexmedetomidine is used for a patient with severe alcohol withdrawal, insist on a regimen of scheduled benzodiazepine such as diazepam 10 mg IV every 6 hours.

Thiamine

Thiamine supplementation is an important part of the treatment of alcohol withdrawal. Thiamine levels are often deficient in patients with alcohol withdrawal. This can lead to the development of Wernicke's Encephalopathy.

IV thiamine for the treatment and prophylaxis of Wernicke's Encephalopathy has generally been considered inexpensive and without significant side effects. For these reasons, organizations such as the Royal College of Physicians in the UK have recommended large IV thiamine doses such as 500 mg q8 hrs for treatment and 250 mg q24 hrs for prophylaxis of Wernicke's Encephalopathy.

REFERENCES

Arch Intern Med. 2002;162(10):1117-1121.
J Trauma and Acute Care Surgery. 2014 Dec;77(6):938–943
Crit Care Med. 2007 Mar; 35(3): 724–730.
Ann Intensive Care. 2012; 2: 12.
Pharmacotherapy. 2014 Sep;34(9):910-7.
Alcohol Alcohol. 2002 Nov-Dec;37(6):513-21.
Ann Pharmacother. 2016 May;50(5):389-401.

Chapter 16

Opioid Overdose

KEY POINTS

1. Life threatening situation? If yes --> Give 0.4 to 2 mg rapid IV push naloxone.

2. Non-life threatening situation? If yes --> Give 0.04 to 0.08 mg naloxone IV every minute until response.

3. Long acting opioid? If yes --> Consider a naloxone infusion. Mix 4 mg naloxone in 100 mL D5W. Starting dose in mg/hour is 2/3 of the dose needed to reverse. Increase by 0.1 to 0.2 mg/hour if respiratory or CNS depression returns.

OBSERVATIONS

Naloxone is a pure opioid antagonist that competes with and displaces opioids at receptor sites. It is useful for reversing respiratory and central nervous system (CNS) depression from opioids. It works within 1 minute and it lasts up to 60 minutes (shorter than the duration of most opioids). Naloxone also immediately precipitates opioid withdrawal, reversing the analgesic effects of opioids.

Prior to giving naloxone ask this question:

Is the patient's life in immediate danger due to opioid effects?

If yes - give large doses of naloxone (the benefit of saving their life outweighs the risk of inducing withdrawal).

If no - titrate smaller doses of naloxone slowly (opioids can be slowly reversed to avoid inducing withdrawal).

INTERVENTIONS

Naloxone dose in life-threatening situations

The goal of naloxone therapy is to immediately reverse the effect of opioids.

Give an initial dose of naloxone 0.4 mg to 2 mg rapid IV push. A dose of 0.4 mg naloxone should be more than enough to reverse therapeutic doses of opioids such as those given to a hospital inpatient.

Patients with massive overdoses of prescription opioids or heroin may require larger doses so it is reasonable to start with 2 mg naloxone for these patients. Although the IV route is preferred, intraosseous, intramuscular, and subcutaneous routes may also be used.

If the initial naloxone dose is partially effective after 1 minute, give the same dose again.

If the initial naloxone dose is ineffective, give a larger dose of naloxone.

At some point if naloxone is not having an effect, the diagnosis of opioid toxicity must be reconsidered:

- If the patient was taking therapeutic doses of opioids and had no response to naloxone after 0.8 mg has been given, other causes of respiratory depression should be considered.

- If the patient is thought to have overdosed on opioids and had no response to naloxone after 10 mg has been given, other causes of respiratory depression should be considered.

A few years ago an elderly patient arrived by ambulance to the Emergency Department comatose and the family reported the patient had an implanted 'pain pump' that was recently refilled. Opioid toxicity was suspected and the patient received a total of 11 mg naloxone with no effect. Supportive care was given and the patient was admitted to the ICU.

It was later discovered the 'pain pump' was an intrathecal baclofen pump and there was a 1,000-fold compounding error made when the pump was refilled. This explained why the patient was comatose and unresponsive to naloxone. The bladder of the pump was drained and replaced with saline, supportive care continued, and the patient recovered without sequelae after a few days.

Scheduled re-dosing or continuous infusions may be necessary in patients likely to experience return of respiratory or CNS depression.

Naloxone dose in non-life-threatening situations

The goal of naloxone therapy is to reverse the respiratory and CNS depressive effects of opioids while maintaining adequate analgesia.

A common scenario for the rapid response team is to be called to a surgical floor to see a patient who does not respond to voice or touch, is breathing at 6-8 breaths per minute with a pulse, and has an O2 saturation of 90%.

Giving 0.4 mg IV push naloxone will almost certainly reverse the respiratory and CNS effects of opioids in a patient like this. But if they just had a major surgery, the patient is likely to experience excruciating pain - and will have to suffer through the duration of action of naloxone before feeling any relief. Such a situation is easily avoided by gradually giving small doses of naloxone and waiting to see the effect. Here is how to do it:

1. Mix 1 mL of 0.4 mg/mL naloxone with 9 mL normal saline in a syringe for IV administration (0.04 mg/mL = 40 mcg/mL).
2. Administer the dilute naloxone solution IV very slowly (1 or 2 mL (40-80 mcg) over 1 minute). Closely observe the patient's response.
3. The patient should open their eyes and respond within 1 to 2 minutes. If not, continue the dilute naloxone solution administration 1 or 2 mL over 1 minute to a total of 20 mL (0.8 mg).

Sometimes, it can be challenging to get the staff in the room to agree to a slow reversal plan rather than a quick one. When this happens emphasize these three points:

1. Because the patient is oxygenating, we have time to reverse them slowly.
2. If the patient is put into withdrawal, we will not be able to treat their pain until the naloxone wears off.
3. Acute withdrawal can precipitate acute agitation and put the staff at risk of being harmed.

Continuous infusion of naloxone

When the opioid effect is expected to be prolonged (massive overdose, methadone, extended release opioid) a continuous infusion of naloxone should be considered. To accomplish this, mix 4 mg naloxone in 100 mL D5W.

The initial infusion rate in mg/hour is 2/3 of the naloxone dose that resulted in reversal of symptoms. For example, if the initial bolus dose which reversed symptoms was 0.8 mg then start the infusion at 0.5 mg/hour.

Titrate the infusion to response: Increase by 0.1 to 0.2 mg/hour if respiratory or CNS depression returns.

Weaning off the naloxone infusion

1. Decrease by 0.1 to 0.2 mg/hour every 2 hours.
2. Assess patient for signs/symptoms of respiratory or CNS depression.
3. If decreased respiratory rate or responsiveness is noted, return to the previous rate and attempt to decrease again in 1 to 2 hours.

The titration or weaning period will vary depending on the duration of action of the opioid and the patient's liver function.

COMPLICATIONS

Monitoring after naloxone is given

The duration of naloxone is shorter than the duration of most opioids. Naloxone may wear off within an hour of administration. The patient should be monitored for 2 hours after giving naloxone for recurrent respiratory or CNS depression. Patients who do not experience respiratory or CNS depression within 2 hours of the last dose of naloxone are not likely to require further doses.

The logistics of getting a naloxone infusion started can sometimes be lengthy. Be prepared to give another dose of naloxone if the infusion is not started immediately.

REFERENCES

Circulation. 2010 Nov;122(18)S3
Emerg Med J. 2005;22:612–616.

Chapter 17

Hypertensive Emergency

KEY POINTS

1. Use IV medications in all instances.

2. Dosing should be based on your local protocols.

3. Treatment choice of hypertensive emergency depends on the cause:

- Ischemic stroke --> Use labetalol or nicardipine
- Hemorrhagic stroke --> Use labetalol or nicardipine
- Head trauma --> Use mannitol
- Hypertensive encephalopathy --> Use nicardipine
- Acute heart failure --> Use loop diuretics and nitroglycerin
- Acute coronary syndrome --> Use nitroglycerin, nicardipine, or esmolol
- Acute aortic dissection --> Use nitroprusside or clevidipine
- Risk to vascular suture lines after vascular surgery --> Use nicardipine or labetalol
- Ingestion of sympathomimetic agents --> Use phentolamine (if available) or nitroprusside
- Pheochromocytoma --> Use nitroprusside, phentolamine, or nicardipine
- Severe autonomic dysfunction --> Use phentolamine (if available) or nitroprusside
- Pregnancy --> Use magnesium sulfate, hydralazine, or labetalol

OBSERVATIONS

A hypertensive emergency is present when severe hypertension is associated with acute, ongoing end-organ damage. Severe hypertension in the absence of end-organ damage used to be called a hypertensive urgency, but is now referred to as acute asymptomatic hypertension. Whether treating a hypertensive emergency or acute asymptomatic hypertension, an excessive hypotensive response is potentially dangerous, and may lead to ischemic complications such as stroke, myocardial infarction, or blindness.

End organ damage is typically found in the form of neurologic, cardiac, vascular, or renal damage.

INTERVENTIONS

The general goal of treatment for most hypertensive emergencies is to achieve a 10-20% reduction in systolic BP in the first hour, and an additional 5-15% reduction in BP in the first 24 hours.

There are two notable exceptions to this general goal:

1. In the acute phase of ischemic stroke, the blood pressure is usually not lowered unless it is ≥185/110 mmHg in patients who are eligible for alteplase therapy or ≥220/120 mmHg in patients who are not eligible for alteplase therapy.
2. In acute aortic dissection, the systolic blood pressure is rapidly lowered to a target of 100 to 120 mmHg within 20 minutes.

The following is a list of each type of hypertensive emergency and the ideal agents to use. Doses should be based on your local protocols.

Neurologic emergencies

The most frequent neurologic hypertensive emergencies are ischemic stroke, hemorrhagic stroke, head trauma, and hypertensive encephalopathy.

Ischemic stroke

Use IV labetalol or nicardipine to achieve a BP <185/110 mmHg if the patient is eligible for alteplase, or <220/120 mmHg if they are not alteplase eligible.

Hemorrhagic stroke

Treatment of acute hypertension in the setting of hemorrhagic stroke is a delicate balance between the risk of reducing cerebral perfusion and the benefit of reduced bleeding. IV labetalol or nicardipine are my preferred medications for these patients.

Head trauma

Hypertension is usually treated in the setting of head trauma only if the cerebral perfusion pressure (mean arterial pressure minus intracranial pressure) is >120 mmHg and the intracranial pressure is >20 mmHg. Use IV mannitol.

Hypertensive encephalopathy

Hypertensive encephalopathy is a diagnosis of exclusion. You will not know the patient had hypertensive encephalopathy until you lower their blood pressure and see their mental status rapidly improve. If you are suspecting hypertensive encephalopathy use IV nicardipine.

Cardiac emergencies

The most frequent cardiac hypertensive emergencies are acute left ventricular dysfunction with pulmonary edema and acute coronary syndrome.

Acute heart failure

Use IV loop diuretics and nitroglycerine. Avoid hydralazine (increases cardiac work) and beta-blockers (decreases cardiac contractility).

Acute coronary syndrome

Use IV nitroglycerin, nicardipine, or esmolol to reduce the underlying coronary ischemia and/or increased myocardial oxygen consumption and to improve outcomes.

Vascular emergencies

The most frequent vascular hypertensive emergencies include acute aortic dissection and risk to suture lines s/p vascular surgery.

Acute aortic dissection

Remember the goal is to lower the systolic blood pressure rapidly to a target of 100 to 120 mmHg within 20 minutes. Use IV nitroprusside or clevidipine.

Risk to vascular suture lines after vascular surgery

I am not aware of any studies comparing agents to use in the scenario of hypertensive emergency s/p vascular surgery. I would use IV nicardipine or labetalol for these patients.

Renal emergencies

Severe hypertension may cause acute hypertensive nephrosclerosis. Antihypertensive therapy often leads to worsening kidney function, sometimes requiring dialysis, although this is sometimes reversible. Fenoldopam, if available, may be a useful antihypertensive in this setting since it is associated with a temporary improvement in renal function.

Other emergencies

Other causes of hypertensive emergencies are sympathetic overactivity and pregnancy.

Sympathetic overactivity may be caused by withdrawal of antihypertensives, ingestion of sympathomimetic agents, pheochromocytoma, or autonomic dysfunction. Unless a beta blocker was recently withdrawn, administration of a beta blocker alone is contraindicated in these settings since inhibition of beta receptor-induced vasodilation can result in unopposed alpha-adrenergic vasoconstriction and a further rise in blood pressure.

Withdrawal of short-acting antihypertensive agents

If the patient is in withdrawal from clonidine, oral clonidine will begin to lower the blood pressure within an hour. This is the only scenario I would use an oral antihypertensive in a hypertensive emergency. Oral beta-blockers are too slow to work. If the patient is in withdrawal from a beta-blocker, other IV antihypertensives should be used while the beta-blocker takes effect.

Ingestion of sympathomimetic agents

Examples of ingested sympathomimetic agents are cocaine, amphetamines, and a tyramine/monoamine oxidase inhibitor interaction. IV phentolamine (if available) or nitroprusside can be used.

Pheochromocytoma

Pheochromocytoma can also produce severe hypertension and acute target-organ damage. Use IV nitroprusside, phentolamine, or nicardipine if a hypertensive emergency presents before adrenalectomy can be performed.

Severe autonomic dysfunction

Acute spinal cord injury or Guillain-Barré syndrome is occasionally associated with hypertensive emergency. Use IV phentolamine (if available) or nitroprusside.

Pregnancy

For hypertensive emergencies during pregnancy use IV magnesium sulfate, hydralazine, or labetalol.

Clevipidine

Clevidipine is not on formulary at my hospital, and I have no experience working with this medication. Looking at the very limited published data on clevidipine, I would be extremely concerned about over-rapid correction of hypertension with clevidipine, and would not consider using it for anything I do not already consider nitroprusside first line for. With the recent price increase of nitroprusside, it looks increasingly likely that clevidipine will make its way onto formulary at my hospital. If you have experience with clevidipine, I would love to hear about it. Send me an email or a voicemail at: pharmacyjoe.com/contact

REFERENCES

Circulation. 1990 Mar;81(3):970-7.
Prog Cardiovasc Dis. 2006 Mar-Apr;48(5):316-25.
Crit Care Med. 2011 Oct;39(10):2330-6.

Chapter 18

Severe Hyperthermia

KEY POINTS

1. Malignant hyperthermia (MH) is extremely rare in the postoperative setting, serotonin syndrome (SS) has a faster onset and neuromuscular hyperactivity, while neuroleptic malignant syndrome (NMS) has a slower onset and neuromuscular hypoactivity.

2. A thorough review of current and recent medications helps to differentiate MH, SS, and NMS.

3. Serotonin syndrome --> Start with 1 or 2 mg of IV lorazepam or midazolam and titrate the dose to effect.

4. Malignant hyperthermia --> Call 800-644-9737 within the US for expert help. Give dantrolene loading dose of 2.5 mg/kg IV, with subsequent bolus doses of 1 mg/kg IV until the signs of acute MH abate. Be prepared for the development of hyperkalemia (see Chapter 21).

5. Neuroleptic malignant syndrome --> Call 607-674-7920 within the US for expert help. Give dantrolene boluses of 1 to 2.5 mg/kg IV and bromocriptine 2.5 mg by mouth or gastric tube every six to eight hour, titrating up to a maximum of 40 mg/day.

OBSERVATIONS

Severe hyperthermia may be caused by serotonin syndrome (SS), malignant hyperthermia (MH), and neuroleptic malignant syndrome (NMS).

Muscular rigidity, significant hyperthermia, and autonomic instability are all common features of serotonin syndrome, malignant hyperthermia, and neuroleptic malignant syndrome. A thorough review of the patient's current and recent medications is the best way to tell the difference between these three conditions.

1. Serotonin syndrome

Serotonin syndrome can result from an overdose or medication interaction involving one or more of the many medications that increase serotonergic activity.

The Hunter Criteria is often used for the diagnosis of serotonin syndrome. To fulfill the Hunter Criteria, a patient must have taken a serotonergic agent and meet ONE of the following conditions:

- Spontaneous clonus
- Inducible clonus PLUS agitation or diaphoresis
- Ocular clonus PLUS agitation or diaphoresis
- Tremor PLUS hyperreflexia
- Hypertonia PLUS temperature above 38°C PLUS ocular clonus or inducible clonus

Serotonin syndrome is very similar to neuroleptic malignant syndrome. A thorough review of the patient's current and recent medications and history of present illness is essential for differentiating between the two syndromes. SS develops over 24 hours; NMS develops over a period of days. SS is accompanied by neuromuscular hyper-reactivity (tremor, hyperreflexia, and myoclonus); NMS is accompanied by sluggish neuromuscular responses (rigidity and bradyreflexia).

Cases of serotonin syndrome that I have seen have included an opioid plus two serotonergic medications. I once encountered a young adult female in my emergency department with confusion, hyperthermia, tachycardia, tremor, hyperreflexia, and diaphoresis. She was on therapeutic doses of citalopram and hydrocodone, but had taken three cyclobenzaprine 10 mg tablets for her severe back pain. The team initially thought she was having an anticholinergic reaction from the extra cyclobenzaprine. I was able to point out that the patient was diaphoretic, so anticholinergic toxicity was unlikely. In addition cyclobenzaprine is a serotonergic agent (in fact it is structurally nearly identical to amitriptyline). We gave the patient cyproheptadine and lorazepam and she recovered quickly.

2. Malignant hyperthermia

Malignant hyperthermia occurs rarely after exposure to halogenated volatile anesthetics and depolarizing muscle relaxants (succinylcholine). Its classic presentation is increased concentrations of end-tidal carbon dioxide, rigor mortis-like muscle rigidity, tachycardia, hyperthermia, and acidosis.

The onset of MH in the postoperative period is extremely rare. Cases thought to be postoperative MH have been described as isolated rhabdomyolysis in otherwise asymptomatic patients, and there is controversy as to whether these represent MH at all.

A great resource that I have called upon many times when MH was in the differential diagnosis is the Malignant Hypethermia Association of the United States (MHAUS). They have a 24/7 hotline (800-644-9737 within the US) for use in emergency situations. Calling the hotline will put you in touch with an expert anesthesiologist within minutes to advise you in selecting the best treatment for the patient.

3. Neuroleptic malignant syndrome

The slow onset of neuroleptic malignant syndrome (mental status changes occurring over one to three days) generally distinguishes it from MH or SS. NMS does not generally occur during administration of general anesthesia. NMS is defined by its association with a class of medications that block dopamine transmission and 4 distinctive findings: fever, rigidity, mental status changes, and autonomic instability.

Medications associated with NMS are the dopamine blocking agents such as neuroleptic medications (haloperidol, olanzapine, etc...) and antiemetics (metoclopramide, droperidol, proclorperazine, and promethazine). NMS is also seen in patients treated for parkinsonism in the setting of withdrawal of levodopa or dopamine agonist therapy, as well as with dose reductions and when switching from one agent to another.

The Neuroleptic Malignant Syndrome Information Service provides an emergency hotline for US medical professionals treating NMS: 607-674-7920.

INTERVENTIONS

Treatment of serotonin syndrome

In addition to supportive care, benzodiazepines are given to eliminate agitation, tremor, clonus, and elevations in heart rate and blood pressure. Start with 1 or 2 mg of IV lorazepam or midazolam and titrate the dose to effect. Cyproheptadine, an anti-serotonergic antihistamine can be given as well. Give 12 mg orally or by orogastric tube as the initial adult dose.

Treatment of malignant hyperthermia

In addition to supportive ventilator strategies, dantrolene should be given immediately to patients with MH. Dantrolene is the only known antidote for MH. It should be administered as a loading dose of 2.5 mg/kg IV, with subsequent bolus doses of 1 mg/kg IV until the signs of acute MH abate. Be prepared for the development of hyperkalemia (see Chapter 21).

Treatment of neuroleptic malignant syndrome

Aggressive supportive care in NMS is essential. It is likely that mechanical ventilation, IV fluids, antihypertensives, and benzodiazepines will be required. Maximally aggressive surface cooling should be used, including cooling blankets and axillary ice packs. The use of endovascular cooling has not been evaluated for the treatment of NMS, but if it was my family member as the patient, I would be pushing hard for this intervention to get their temperature down.

Recommended treatments for NMS are based upon case reports and clinical experience, not upon data from clinical trials. Commonly recommended medications are dantrolene, bromocriptine, and amantadine. Their use is controversial and largely unsupported. However due to lack of other proven treatments and high morbidity and mortality of the disorder, it is likely one or more of these medications will be requested for a patient who develops NMS.

Dantrolene

Dantrolene doses of 1 to 2.5 mg/kg IV are typically used and can be repeated to a maximum dose of 10 mg/kg/day. Efficacy includes reduction of heat production and rigidity, and effects are reported within minutes of administration. The duration of treatment required is unclear, with recommendations ranging from a few to 10 days of treatment.

Bromocriptine

Bromocriptine, a dopamine agonist, is given to restore lost dopaminergic tone. Start with 2.5 mg by mouth or gastric tube every six to eight hours and titrate up to a maximum of 40 mg/day. Continue bromocriptine for 10 days after NMS is controlled and then taper slowly.

Amantadine

Amantadine has dopaminergic and anticholinergic effects and is used as an alternative to bromocriptine. The starting dose is 100 mg by mouth or gastric tube and is titrated upward as needed to a maximum of 200 mg every 12 hours.

REFERENCES

QJM. 2003 Aug;96(9):635-642
mhaus.org
Crit Care. 2007; 11(1): R4.
Brain Res. 1996 Dec 16;743(1-2):263-70.

Chapter 19

Hypoglycemia

KEY POINTS

1. Treatment of hypoglycemia should occur as quickly as possible to prevent neurologic injury.

2. If the patient can take oral glucose, give 20 grams of oral glucose gel/tablets or 4 ounces of orange or apple juice.

3. If the patient has IV access, give 50 mL of 50% dextrose (25 g) rapid IV push.

4. If the patient does not have oral or IV access, give glucagon 1mg IM.

OBSERVATIONS

Hypoglycemia is a common reason for activation of in-hospital rapid response teams. It constitutes a medical emergency, however most individuals will recover completely with treatment.

Hypoglycemia may range from a mild lowering of glucose (< 70 mg/dL) with minimal or no symptoms to severe hypoglycemia (< 40 mg/dL) and neurological symptoms.

The lack of ATP generation results in both adrenergic and CNS responses, which comprise the symptoms of hypoglycemia.

Adrenergic signs and symptoms of hypoglycemia

The adrenergic signs and symptoms of hypoglycemia include anxiety, irritability, dizziness, diaphoresis, pallor, tachycardia, headache, shakiness, and hunger.

CNS signs and symptoms of hypoglycemia

The CNS signs and symptoms of hypoglycemia include altered mental status that proceeds to headache, malaise, impaired concentration, confusion, disorientation, irritability, lethargy, slurred speech, and irrational or uncontrolled behavior.

More serious CNS effects include seizures and hemiplegia.

At a blood glucose level of 10 mg/dL hypoglycemia manifests as coma, pupillary dilation, shallow breathing, bradycardia, and hypotonicity.

When responding to any in-hospital rapid response call where an adrenergic sign of hypoglycemia or altered mental status is present, a fingerstick blood glucose value should be checked immediately.

Causes of Hypoglycemia

Common causes of hypoglycemia in the inpatient setting are:

- Medication effect (usually insulin or other hypoglycemics)
- Antidiabetic medication use without appropriate carbohydrate intake
- Critical illness such as major organ failure, sepsis, and severe trauma

Rare causes of hypoglycemia include:

- Endocrine disorders
- Tumors
- Ingestion of large amounts of alcohol or salicylates
- Sudden reduction of corticosteroid dose
- Emesis
- Reduction of rate of intravenous dextrose
- Interruption of enteral feedings or parenteral nutrition
- Medication error

INTERVENTIONS

Treatment of hypoglycemia should occur as quickly as possible to prevent neurologic injury.

The two decision points in treatment are:

1. Whether the patient can take oral glucose
2. Whether the patient has IV access

In patients with hypoglycemia who can take oral glucose, 20 grams of glucose should be administered. If glucose gel or tablets are not immediately accessible, 4 ounces of orange or apple juice can be used.

In patients with hypoglycemia who are unable to take oral glucose, IV access should be established and 50 mL of 50% dextrose (25 g) should be administered rapidly.

In patients with hypoglycemia who are unable to take oral glucose and are without IV access, glucagon 1mg IM should be administered immediately.

Glucagon

Glucagon stimulates adenylate cyclase to produce increased cyclic AMP. This promotes hepatic glycogenolysis and gluconeogenesis causing blood glucose levels to increase. This antihypoglycemic effect is dependent upon preexisting hepatic glycogen stores.

Extra hepatic effects of glucagon include relaxation of the smooth muscle of the stomach, duodenum, small bowel, and colon.

Nausea and vomiting from glucagon is rare when used at a dose of 1mg IM.

After treatment

Once the hypoglycemia is treated, efforts should be made to evaluate and treat the underlying cause. A thorough review of recent and current medications is essential to this process.

Blood glucose should be rechecked 15 minutes after the first intervention. Additional blood glucose monitoring should be done depending on the cause of hypoglycemia.

Antidote to sulfonylurea induced hypoglycemia

If the cause of hypoglycemia is due to a sulfonylurea, an antidote is available. Sulfonylureas work by stimulating insulin release from the pancreatic beta cells and reducing glucose output from the liver.

A direct antidote to sulfonylureas is octreotide. Octreotide mimics natural somatostatin by inhibiting the release of serotonin, gastrin,

VIP, insulin, glucagon, secretin, motilin, and pancreatic polypeptide.

Usually, patients with hypoglycemia from sulfonylureas will have recurrent episodes of severe hypoglycemia until the sulfonylurea is cleared. Giving a subcutaneous dose of 50 to 100 mcg octreotide can stop the insulin release caused by sulfonylureas and stabilize the patient's blood glucose.

REFERENCES

Diabetes Spectrum. 2005 Jan; 18(1): 39-44.
http://pi.lilly.com/us/rglucagon-pi.pdf
J Med Toxicol. 2010 Jun;6(2):199-206.
Crit Care. 2005; 9(6): 543–549.

Chapter 20

Hyponatremia from SIADH

KEY POINTS

1. For severe hyponatremia, give a 100 mL bolus of 3 percent saline, and repeat this once or twice if neurologic symptoms persist or worsen.

2. Avoid normal saline as this will worsen hyponatremia in syndrome of inappropriate antidiuretic hormone (SIADH).

3. If during correction of hyponatremia serum sodium rises greater than 9 mEq in 24 hours (or 18 mEq in 48 hrs), consider re-lowering of the serum sodium to avoid permanent neurologic damage:

- Give boluses of 6mL/kg of 5% dextrose in water IV, repeated until the serum sodium rise is back below 9 mEq in 24 hours (or 18 mEq in 48 hours)
- In addition give desmopressin 2 mcg every 6 hours IV or subcutaneously

OBSERVATIONS

SIADH stands for Syndrome of Inappropriate Anti-Diuretic Hormone. In this syndrome, there is too much antidiuretic hormone in circulation. Anti-diuretic hormone promotes water retention and solute loss in the collecting duct of the nephron. Too much ADH, and you end up with too much water retention and solute loss. The solute that is lost is primarily sodium, and this combined with excess water retention is what leads to hyponatremia in SIADH.

SIADH can be caused by CNS damage or CNS disorders, cancer, lung disease, and medications. The list of medications that have been associated with causing SIADH is long. The most common medication classes that cause SIADH in patients are antiepileptics, antipsychotics, and antidepressants.

Symptoms vary with the duration and severity of hyponatremia. Hyponatremia from SIADH can often be severe - with a sodium 120 mEq/L or lower. Patients may present with seizure or coma at this level if the hyponatremia is acute.

Mild to moderate symptoms of hyponatremia are relatively nonspecific and include headache, nausea, vomiting, fatigue, gait disturbances, and confusion. In patients with more acute hyponatremia, such symptoms could rapidly change without warning to seizures, respiratory arrest, and herniation.

INTERVENTIONS

In addition to stopping potentially causative medications, there are two main treatment strategies for the acute treatment of SIADH:

1. Fluid restriction
2. Sodium chloride

Vasopressin receptor antagonists are a potential third option. They are not covered here since they have not been adequately studied for the initial treatment of acute hyponatremia from SIADH.

Fluid restriction

Fluid restriction with a goal intake of less than 800 mL/day should be considered in all patients with hyponatremia from SIADH. This may be all that is necessary if the patient has mild-moderate symptoms or has severe hyponatremia without symptoms.

The effectiveness of fluid restriction alone can be predicted by the urine to serum cation ratio. A ratio less than 0.5 suggests that the serum sodium concentration will rise with fluid restriction, while a ratio greater than 1 indicates that it will not. Interestingly, if this ratio is greater than 1, loop diuretics will be effective in increasing water loss and raising the serum sodium concentration.

In addition to fluid restriction, the therapy of SIADH-associated hyponatremia often requires the administration of sodium chloride, either as oral salt tablets or intravenous saline.

Sodium chloride

Oral salt tablets can be used in patients with mild to moderate hyponatremia.

When using intravenous saline, the electrolyte concentration of the administered fluid must be greater than the electrolyte concentration of the urine. This usually requires the use of hypertonic saline.

If a patient has severe symptomatic hyponatremia including seizures or other severe neurologic abnormalities or intracerebral diseases, IV hypertonic saline should be given immediately. Give a 100 mL bolus of 3 percent saline, and repeat this once or twice if neurologic symptoms persist or worsen.

In an ideal situation, hypertonic saline would be given via a central line.

Any (IV) port in a storm.

The priority is to fix the neurologic disorder - IV access can be optimized after the hypertonic saline has been started.

Why normal saline makes SIADH worse

On the surface, it is easy to think that giving normal saline (154 mEq/L) to a patient with hyponatremia from SIADH will help raise the serum sodium. But in the case of SIADH, giving normal saline will actually lower the serum sodium even more. Here is why:

Sodium and water handling by the kidney are regulated independently: sodium by aldosterone and atrial natriuretic peptide; and water by ADH. In SIADH, sodium handling is intact and only water handling is out of balance from too much ADH. Therefore when administering 1 liter of normal saline to a patient with SIADH and a high urine osmolality, all of the sodium will be excreted but about half of the water will be retained. This will result in worsening hyponatremia. This is because the concentration of sodium in the urine of a patient with SIADH is going to be higher than the concentration of sodium in normal saline.

With sodium handling by aldosterone intact, in order to raise the serum sodium with IV fluids, the sodium concentration of the administered IV fluids must be greater than the concentration of sodium in the urine - not the serum.

COMPLICATIONS

What to do if you raise the sodium too high too fast

After the neurologic symptoms are under control, further calculations can be performed to determine how much sodium chloride the patient still needs. Ideally, the serum sodium will not rise by more than 4 to 6 mEq in the first 24 hours of treatment.

This target is lower than I remember learning in pharmacy school, but a lower target provides a better margin of safety should the sodium rise too fast.

The risk of correcting the serum sodium concentration too quickly is osmotic demyelination of the nervous system. This syndrome results in irreversible or partially reversible neurologic damage.

The risk is serious enough that if a patient with hyponatremia has a serum sodium rise greater than 9 mEq in 24 hours (or 18 mEq in 48 hrs), re-lowering of the serum sodium should be considered. This is supported by animal data which show effectiveness in preventing osmotic demyelination syndrome.

The regimen to use is 6mL/kg of 5% dextrose in water IV, repeated until the serum sodium rise is back below 9 mEq in 24 hours (or 18 mEq in 48 hours). Desmopressin also is given at a dose of 2 mcg every 6 hours IV or subcutaneously.

REFERENCES

Indian J Endocrinol Metab. 2014 Nov-Dec; 18(6): 760–771.
J Am Soc Nephrol. 2008 Jun;19(6):1054-8.

Chapter 21

Hyperkalemia

KEY POINTS

1. Give calcium chloride 1 g IV push

2. Give regular insulin 10 units IV push

3. Give dextrose 25 g IV push

4. Consider hemodialysis

5. Check ECG for signs of improvement

6. Check fingerstick glucose 1 hour after insulin

7. Check for medication related causes of hyperkalemia

OBSERVATIONS

Severe hyperkalemia can be recognized by:

- Cardiac conduction abnormalities on ECG (Flattened P waves , Widened QRS interval, or Peaked T waves)

- Muscle weakness or paralysis

- Serum potassium value greater than 7 mEq / L

An ECG from a patient with a serum potassium of 7.5 with flattened P waves, widened QRS interval, and peaked T waves:

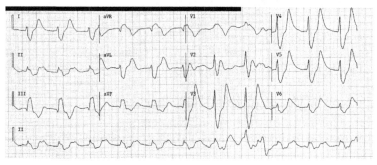

Courtesy of R.W. Koster, MD, PhD, The Netherlands   ECG ЭPEDIA.ORG

In a patient without chronically high potassium, a value lower than 7 may still have severe consequences.

INTERVENTIONS

Treatment of severe hyperkalemia should follow a three step process:

1. Protect the cardiac membrane with IV calcium
2. Hide the potassium from the heart with insulin and dextrose
3. Remove the excess potassium from the patient

Protect the cardiac membrane with IV calcium

Give calcium chloride 1g rapid IV push OR calcium gluconate 2g IV over 15 minutes.

Calcium chloride can be given IV push, but causes a significant amount of phlebitis and tissue injury in extravasation. Therefore calcium chloride is best used if there is a life threatening arrhythmia present or a central line is in place.

Calcium gluconate is less potent and causes less irritation. It must be given at a slower rate of 150 mg/minute to avoid hypotension. Calcium gluconate is best used if the patient has a small, peripheral IV line and can tolerate waiting ~15 minutes for the dose to infuse.

Hide the potassium from the heart with insulin and dextrose

Give 10 units IV push regular insulin AND 25 to 50 grams dextrose IV push.

Insulin forces potassium inside cells, temporarily 'hiding' it away from the cardiac membranes. The intracellular concentrations of sodium and potassium are essentially the reverse of the plasma concentrations. This is why a couple extra mEq/L of potassium does not do any harm inside cells, but has a tremendous impact on the outside of cells.

Even if the patient is already hyperglycemic, some IV dextrose should be given to ensure hypoglycemia does not develop. In this case it may be reasonable to give 25 grams of dextrose instead of 50.

Nebulized albuterol and IV sodium bicarbonate are not practical treatments for acute hyperkalemia.

Remove the excess potassium from the patient

For severe hyperkalemia the treatment of choice to remove excess potassium is hemodialysis.

Sodium polystyrene sulfate (SPS) is a cation exchange resin. The best evidence available suggests that this medication is no more effective than laxative use for lowering serum potassium levels.

Sodium polystyrene sulfate is often considered for the treatment of acute hyperkalemia. While not common, sodium polystyrene sulfate can cause intestinal necrosis, a potentially fatal complication. Certain conditions lead to a higher incidence of intestinal necrosis from SPS and should be considered absolute contraindications to use:

- Postoperative patients
- Patients with an ileus or who are receiving opioids
- Patients with a bowel obstruction

COMPLICATIONS

If the patient's cardiac rhythm or general appearance worsens, make sure preparations for cardiac arrest are readily available.

Check a fingerstick blood glucose 1 hour after insulin / dextrose administration.

If hemodialysis is not readily available, and the patient has a contraindication to SPS, use bolus or continuous infusions of insulin and dextrose until arrangements for dialysis can be made.

Ensure that the order of treatment is correctly prioritized (calcium before insulin).

REFERENCES

ecgpedia.org
Crit Care Med. 2008 Dec;36(12):3246-51.
J Am Soc Nephrol. 2010 May;21(5):733-5.
Kidney Int. 1992 Feb;41(2):369-74.

Will You Do Me a Favor?

If you have found *A Pharmacists Guide to Inpatient Medical Emergencies* helpful, would you mind taking a moment to write a review on Amazon? Even a short review will help others discover this book.

If someone you know would find this book helpful, please tell them about it or send them a copy.

Finally, if you would like to get the free bonus materials discussed throughout this book, you can signup at pharmacyjoe.com/bonus.

Stay Connected

Tune in to hear Pharmacy Joe's #1 ranked critical care pharmacy podcast: The Elective Rotation. On the podcast you will hear concise, unbiased episodes about current topics in critical care pharmacy.

You can find the show in iTunes, Stitcher, or by going to pharmacyjoe.com.

You can connect with Pharmacy Joe here:

Twitter: pharmacyjoe.com/Twitter
LinkedIn: pharmacyjoe.com/LinkedIn
Website: pharmacyjoe.com/Contact

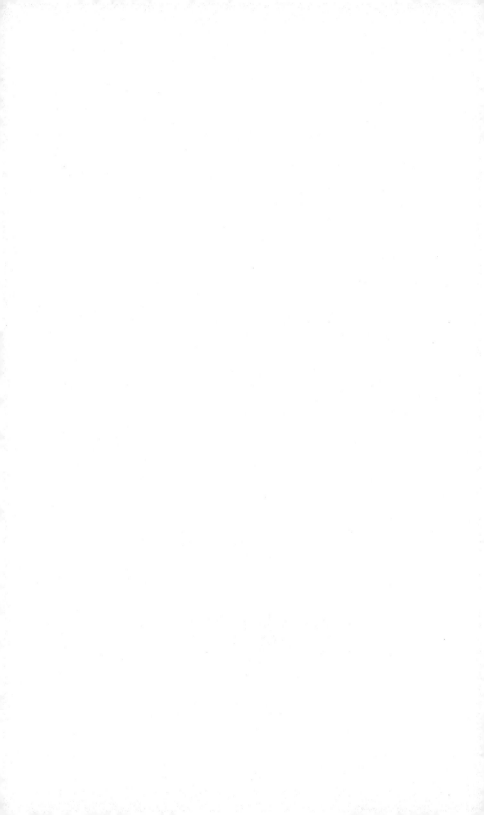

Made in the USA
Middletown, DE
13 June 2023